Case Analysis in Clinical Ethics

Case Analysis in Clinical Ethics is a grounded review from a team of leading ethicists covering the main methods for analysing ethical problems in modern medicine. Anneke Lucassen, a clinician, begins by presenting an ethically challenging genetics case drawn from her clinical experience. It is then analysed from different theoretical points of view. Each ethicist takes a particular approach, illustrating it in action and giving the reader a basic grounding in its central elements. Each chapter can be read on its own, but comparison between them gives the reader a sense of how far methodology in medical ethics matters, and how different theoretical starting points can lead to different practical conclusions. At the end, Dr Lucassen gives a clinician's response to the various ethical methods described.

Practising clinical ethicists and students on upper level undergraduate and Master's degree courses in medical ethics and applied philosophy will find this invaluable.

Richard Ashcroft is head of the Medical Ethics Unit in the Faculty of Medicine at Imperial College London.

Anneke Lucassen is a consultant in clinical genetics at the Wessex Clinical Genetics Service and Senior Lecturer at Southampton University.

Michael Parker is Professor of Bioethics and Director of the Ethox Centre at the University of Oxford.

Marian Verkerk is Professor of Ethics and Care in the Medical Faculty of the University of Groningen.

Guy Widdershoven is Professor of Ethics of Healthcare at the University of Maastricht.

Case Analysis in Clinical Ethics

Edited by

Richard Ashcroft, Anneke Lucassen

Michael Parker, Marian Verkerk

Guy Widdershoven

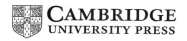

CAMBRIDGE
UNIVERSITY PRESS

CAMBRIDGE UNIVERSITY PRESS
Cambridge, New York, Melbourne, Madrid, Cape Town, Singapore, São Paulo

CAMBRIDGE UNIVERSITY PRESS
The Edinburgh Building, Cambridge CB2 2RU, UK

Published in the United States of America by Cambridge University Press, New York

www.cambridge.org
Information on this title: www.cambridge.org/9780521835497

First published 2005

Printed in the United Kingdom at the University Press, Cambridge

A record for this book is available from the British Library

Library of Congress in Publication data

ISBN-13 978-0-521-83549-7 hardback
ISBN-10 0-521-83549-6 hardback
ISBN-13 978-0-521-54315-6 paperback
ISBN-10 0-521-54315-0 paperback

This book is dedicated to Louise Sarch

Contents

Notes on contributors

George Agich

George J. Agich Ph.D. is Professor in the Cleveland Clinic Lerner College of Medicine and the F. J. O'Neill Chair in Clinical Bioethics at The Cleveland Clinic Foundation (CCF). He directs the CCF Ethics Consultation Service providing over 200 consultations annually. George is the author of many articles and books on a wide range of topics in bioethics and philosophy of medicine. Recent papers have dealt with ethics consultation, bioethics expert testimony, philosophical aspects of psychiatric nosology, ageing and autonomy in long-term care. His most recent book, *Dependence and Autonomy in Long Term Care*, was published by Cambridge University Press in 2003. His current research includes questions of authority, justification and methodology in ethics consultation as well as the ethics of innovation in medicine and surgery.

Richard Ashcroft

Richard Ashcroft is Leverhulme Senior Lecturer in Medical Ethics and Head of the Medical Ethics Unit at Imperial College London. He was previously Lecturer in Ethics in Medicine at Bristol University, where he is still an honorary Research Fellow, and has done research at the Universities of Cambridge and Liverpool. His principal research interests are in ethics of medical research and genetics. He is a member of the UK Gene Therapy Advisory Committee. As well as his respectable interests in practical medical ethics, he has a longstanding interest in continental philosophy and social theory. His contributions to this book are part of his continuing attempt to bring these interests together.

Alastair Campbell

Alastair Campbell is Professor Emeritus of Ethics in Medicine in the School of Medicine, University of Bristol, and Director of the Centre for Ethics in Medicine. He is a former President of the International Association of Bioethics. Recent publications include *Health as Liberation* (1995) and *Medical Ethics*, co-authored with Max Charlesworth, Grant Gillett and Gareth Jones (2001). Professor Campbell is a member of the Medical Ethics Committee of the British Medical Association and a former member of the

Ethics Committee of the Royal College of Obstetricians and Gynaecologists. He served on the Minister of Health's Review Team into the arrangements for surrogacy in the UK and, more recently, as a member of the Chief Medical Officer's Expert Group on Cloning. Professor Campbell is currently Chairman of the Wellcome Trust's Standing Advisory Group on Ethics and Vice-chairman of the Retained Organs Commission. In 1999 he was awarded the Henry K. Beecher Award of the Hastings Center (jointly with Raanan Gillon).

Raanan Gillon

Raanan Gillon is Emeritus Professor of Medical Ethics at Imperial College London where he still does some post-retirement lecturing, teaching and research. He was part-time senior partner in the British National Health Service general practice based at Imperial College London until he retired at the end of 2002. He was editor for 20 years of the *Journal of Medical Ethics* until he retired from that in 2001. He is currently Chairman of the Institute of Medical Ethics and Deputy Chairman of the British Medical Association's Medical Ethics Committee. He has published extensively in the area of medical ethics, and his series of 26 articles in the *British Medical Journal* in the 1980s continues to be reprinted as a small volume, *Philosophical Medical Ethics*, published by Wiley. In 1999 he was awarded the Henry K. Beecher Award of the Hastings Center (jointly with Alastair Campbell).

Søren Holm

Søren Holm B.A., M.A., M.D., Ph.D., Dr.Med.Sci. is Professorial Fellow in Bioethics at the Cardiff Law School and the Cardiff Institute of Society, Health and Ethics, and Professor of Medical Ethics at the Centre for Medical Ethics, University of Oslo. He is a medical doctor and philosopher and has written extensively on moral decision-making. Among his most recent publications is Søren Holm and Monique Jonas, eds., *Engaging the World: The Use of Empirical Research in Bioethics and the Regulation of Biotechnology* (2004).

Brian Hurwitz

Brian Hurwitz holds the D'Oyly Carte Chair of Medicine and the Arts at King's College London. He studied medicine and history and philosophy of science at Cambridge, completed his clinical education in London and commenced in general practice in 1985. His research interests encompass clinical medicine, ethics, medical law and narrative studies in relation to clinical work. Books include *Clinical Guidelines and the Law* (1998), *Narrative-Based Medicine: Dialogue and Discourse in Clinical Practice* (with P. Greenhalgh (eds.), 1998), *NICE, CHI and the NHS Reforms* (with A. Miles and J. Hampton (eds.), 2000), *Clinical Governance* (with A. Miles and

A. Hill (eds.), 2001) and *Narrative Research in Health and Illness* (with P. Greenhalgh and V. Skultans (eds.), 2004). He continues to work as an NHS GP.

Anneke Lucassen

Anneke Lucassen is a senior lecturer/consultant in clinical genetics at the Wessex Clinical Genetics Service and Senior Lecturer at Southampton University. She has a longstanding research interest in the ethical and social issues related both to research and clinical developments in genetics. She is involved with several primary care genetics research projects and has co-authored a book on genetics and primary care. She is a member of her local research-ethics committee and the hospital clinical ethics committee, which are increasingly asked to discuss issues related to genetics. Together with others she has founded and runs the Genethics Club a national forum which meets several times a year for the discussion of ethico-legal issues encountered in the working lives of clinical genetics professionals (http://www.genethicsclub.org).

Michael Parker

Michael Parker is Professor of Bioethics and Director of the Ethox Centre at the University of Oxford and Honorary Clinical Ethicist at the Oxford Radcliffe Hospitals Trust, providing ethics support and education in the clinical setting, particularly in clinical genetics. As Director of the Oxford Genetics and Society Research Programme, he is leading the ethical, legal, psychological, economics and social science programme of the Oxford Genetics Knowledge Park. Mike is Associate Editor of the *Journal of Medical Ethics*, a member of the Board of the International Association of Bioethics, a member of the ethics committee of the Royal College of Physicians and a member of the steering committee of the UK Clinical Ethics Network. His main research interests are in the ethical and social implications of biotechnology, and ethical issues in the clinical genetics setting. He is the author, with Donna Dickenson, of the *Cambridge Medical Ethics Workbook* (Cambridge University Press, 2001).

Julian Savulescu

Julian Savulescu is Uehiro Chair in Practical Ethics at the University of Oxford. He is the Founder and Director of the Oxford Uehiro Centre for Practical Ethics. The Centre is devoted to research, education and stimulating open public discussion around the ethical issues which arise in everyday life and which are related to the changes in society, particularly related to technological advancement. He is also Head of the Melbourne–Oxford Stem Cell Collaboration, devoted to examining the ethical implications of cloning and embryonic stem-cell research. He holds an honorary professorial position at the University of Melbourne, Australia, at the Murdoch Children's Research Institute, Royal Children's Hospital. He was editor of the prestigious *Journal of Medical Ethics* from 2001 to 2004. Previously, he was Director of the Ethics of Genetics Unit at the Murdoch Children's Research Institute. He was also Director of the Bioethics Program at the Centre for the Study of Health and Society at the University of Melbourne and was the Chair of the Department of Human Services, Victoria, Ethics Committee. He has made over 150 presentations and over 150 media appearances (including print, radio and television). Julian is qualified in medicine, bioethics and analytic philosophy. He is author (with Tony Hope and Judith Hendrick) of a textbook for medical students – *Medical Ethics and Law: The Core Curriculum*. He has worked as Clinical Ethicist at the Oxford Radcliffe Hospitals.

Marian Verkerk

Marian Verkerk has studied philosophy. In 1985 she published her thesis on ethics and welfare policy. As a senior lecturer on ethics she has worked at the University of Utrecht and the Erasmus University in Rotterdam. In 1995 she received a Socrates Professorship on Ethics of Care at the University of Groningen. Since 2001 she has been full Professor in Ethics and Care at the Faculty of Medicine of the University of Groningen and the Groningen University Hospital. She is also head of the Expertise Centre of Ethics of Care at the Groningen University Hospital. This centre specialises in ethical consultancy and ethical training for professionals. Marian Verkerk is member of one of the regional review committees on euthanasia and physician-assisted suicide. She is a member of the standing committee of Medical Ethics and Health Law of the Health Council in the Netherlands. She is chair of the Netherlands Association of Bioethics. Marian frequently publishes on issues of ethics, care, care for the chronically ill and psychiatry. One of the most recent subjects of research is on the 'reflective professional'.

Guy Widdershoven

Guy Widdershoven is Professor of Ethics of Health Care at the University of Maastricht. His main theoretical interest is in hermeneutic ethics (focusing on deliberative approaches to decision-making) and ethics of care (emphasising relational autonomy). He supervises research projects on ethics of chronic care (care for the elderly, psychiatry and care for people with a mental disability). He is also involved in projects on ethical aspects of care around the end of life, particularly palliative care and euthanasia. Currently he is scientific director of Caphri (Care and Public Health Research Institute, Maastricht University). He is also President of EACME (European Association of Centres of Medical Ethics).

Rob Withers

Dr Rob Withers has held senior posts in higher education, including Principal of University College Scarborough. He is an occasional visiting lecturer and external examiner and writes fiction and academic articles.

Acknowledgements

The editors would like to thank NWO Geesteswetenschappen for an International Research Grant, which made possible the workshops that were an essential element in the development of this book. They would also like to thanks the Netherlands School for Research in Practical Philosophy and to thank Annemieke Brouwers for the good care she took of us all during the two workshops in the Netherlands.

Richard Ashcroft would like to record his thanks to Guy for the original idea, to Marian for getting the money that supported the project, to Mike for the momentum, to the contributors for contributing, and to Anneke for putting up with us philosophers. Thanks also to Pauline Graham for her constant support at Cambridge University Press.

Michael Parker would like to thank the Universities of Maastricht and Groningen for visiting professorships in 2003 that allowed him to work on preparing the book for submission to the publishers.

Philosophical introduction: case analysis in clinical ethics

Richard Ashcroft, Michael Parker, Marian Verkerk, Guy Widdershoven

Medical ethics has had a rich and complex history over the past 40 years. It has been transformed from a rather clear and straightforward set of rules and attitudes, shaped largely by the medical profession itself, into a major field of academic and social inquiry. Contemporary work in medical ethics can be divided into three parts: ethical analysis and arguments of large-scale issues in science, practice and policy (such as consideration of the ethical issues concerning cloning or resource allocation); theoretical inquiry into the foundations of medical ethics; and practical analysis of particular dilemmas in clinical practice. This last area in medical ethics is normally referred to as clinical ethics, and is in many respects the most important and vibrant part of medical ethics today. It lives through its intimate connection with clinical practice and medical and healthcare education, the ways in which suggestions made by practitioners of clinical ethics are rapidly tested in clinical reality, and the growth of a practical field of work in which 'ethicists' support patients, professionals and ethics committees in making good decisions in difficult circumstances.

For all this vibrant growth, there has been some unease with the way clinical ethics has developed. Healthcare professionals are sometimes baffled by the argumentative curlicues of the philosophers; patients and activists are often suspicious that all this 'ethics' is just a way of reinforcing existing professional attitudes and authority, and that ethicists are just as blind to patients' concerns as the medical professionals; and philosophers are generally infuriated by the apparent laziness and lack of rigour of their 'applied' colleagues. What most of the critics of contemporary clinical ethics agree on is the way in which clinical ethics seems to have become excessively simplified, giving the impression that ethical thinking in clinical situations is a routine and mechanical business, which collapses into a vulgar utilitarianism or an obsession with autonomy as a master value, taking precedence over any other concern. While this is a grotesque parody of the best work in practical and theoretical clinical ethics, it is a picture that is uncomfortably

Case Analysis in Clinical Ethics, ed. Richard Ashcroft, Anneke Lucassen, Michael Parker, Marian Verkerk, Guy Widdershoven. Published by Cambridge University Press.

familiar to anyone who has been involved in the teaching of students, professionals or ethics committee members in the elements of clinical ethics.

In recent years, this situation has led periodically to debates over method in clinical ethics. A particularly important debate took place in the early 1990s over the respective merits of 'principlist' ethics in the tradition of Thomas Beauchamp and James Childress's seminal *Principles of Biomedical Ethics*, and of casuistry, as revived most notably in Albert Jonsen and Stephen Toulmin's *The Abuse of Casuistry*. Other important contributions to enriching clinical ethics came from European philosophy, especially in the phenomenological tradition, exemplified by Richard Zaner's *Ethics and the Clinical Encounter*. There was a considerable body of work that focused on the analysis of meaning and narrative, as a reaction to the highly abstract case reports usually used as the 'data' of clinical ethics; this work was typified by Howard Brody's *Stories of Sickness* and Kathryn Montgomery Hunter's *Doctors' Stories*. Important contributions were made in the various feminist traditions, such as the ethics-of-care tradition springing from Carol Gilligan's *In a Different Voice*, or from the political feminism of Susan Sherwin's *No Longer Patient*. Finally, there was a strong upsurge of interest in 'virtue-ethical' approaches to thinking about problems from the point of view of the character and motivation of participants in moral decision-making, of which Rosalind Hursthouse's *Beginning Lives* was a particularly fine example.

Just as in clinical ethics, within mainstream moral philosophy there was a growing frustration with standard utilitarian and Kantian approaches to normative and applied ethics, as well as a search for post-Marxist alternatives to Rawlsian liberal political philosophy. This led to a growth in moral philosophising within the European tradition, both by active philosophers within that tradition (Lévinas, Derrida, Lyotard, Deleuze, Ricoeur Gadamer and Habermas), and by English-language writers influenced by these currents in European thought. Interestingly, many of these writers took a specific interest in medicine and healthcare, publishing books or articles contributing to debates over the doctor–patient relationship, the meaning of death, and biotechnology and eugenics. This rather gave the lie to the claim that European moral philosophy since Kant had not been practical in orientation (with the clear exception of existentialism). Nevertheless, a characteristic of much of this writing seemed to be that while it could deepen and enrich our understanding of the nature of the problems faced by doctors and patients, this same emphasis on understanding (and its inevitable gaps) undermined any possibility of deriving practical recommendations about what to do.

The origins of the present book lie in a session organised by Guy Widdershoven at the International Association of Bioethics 5th World Congress in Tokyo in November 1998. Guy invited Marian Verkerk, Michael Parker and George Agich to prepare discussions of Simone de Beauvoir's *A Very Easy Death*, which would illustrate how the philosophical methodologies favoured by each contributor could produce illuminating readings and critiques of this famous autobiographical account of de Beauvoir's mother's highly medicalised death. Guy and his colleagues felt that while there was considerable interest in 'European' philosophical methods, there was a good deal of misunderstanding about what these consisted of, what they could achieve, and how far they converged or diverged from each other and from the 'mainstream' principlist and utilitarian methods of English-language bioethics. Somewhat at the last minute Richard Ashcroft was invited to chair the session, and subsequently Guy and Richard decided to edit the papers for publication. Over the next few months it became clear that the idea of a comparative presentation and analysis of different alternatives to principlism and utilitarianism had much more potential, and it was decided to extend the range of contributions, and to produce a book. Michael and Marian were invited to join the editorial team, and a grant in aid of the preparation of the book was obtained from the Dutch Academy of Sciences.

It was decided that organising the book around de Beauvoir's book had various disadvantages, not least the length of her book and the difficulties we would face in reproducing substantial portions of it and in asking new contributors to spend a considerable amount of time reading and analysing it. More importantly, her book could no longer be taken to be an accurate reflection of contemporary approaches to caring for dying patients. We decided to organise the book around a contemporary case. Feeling that many of the most interesting issues arise in clinical genetics, we invited Anneke Lucassen, a geneticist colleague of Mike's with an established interest in ethics, to prepare a case report based on her own and her colleagues' clinical experience. The features of the case report we looked for were: that it should be described in detail with as much richness as possible in characterisation and narrative complexity, to enable close and critical reading and to convey a sense of the difficulties facing the practising clinician in real world practice; that the case should be, as far as possible, a 'normally difficult' case rather than some out of the way once-in-a-lifetime dilemma; that the scientific aspects should be reasonably stable in terms of how genetics was developing (so that while some details could go out of date, the nature of the moral dilemma would remain commonplace for the coming few years); and that the dilemmas faced in genetics would be reasonably recognisable to clinicians and others not working in genetics (for instance, that the issues of family practice would be reasonably familiar to primary care physicians or paediatricians).

The contributors were invited to write commentaries on the case that illustrated the philosophical approach selected, and that came to practical conclusions. Our interest was specifically in whether a given philosophical approach could do more than simply give an interesting redescription of the case and its ethical issues. We wanted to know whether different methods were attuned to different ethical issues, whether they evaluated different factors differently or with different weighting, and whether – aside from differences en route to the 'answer' – they tended to agree on their conclusions or whether they diverged. In this sense the writing of the book was an exercise in experimental practical philosophy. Does it actually matter which method one uses? Or are some methods better for some purposes? How far are conclusions constrained by the method used, how far by presuppositions independent of method about goals and values of medicine such as respect for confidentiality, and how far by values of the writers themselves?

All of the contributors were invited to write because of their recognised status as leaders in biomedical and clinical ethics or moral philosophy, and because of their preference, in their written and clinical work, for using the method we invited them to discuss. Everyone is to that extent a partisan and proponent of the method they discuss. Each contributor was invited to one of a series of four meetings, held in Oxford, Maastricht, Groningen and London, where they would present their chapter draft, and it would be discussed with them in a seminar by the editors, other contributors, and passing graduate students, after which they would return home and revise the chapter in the light of the discussion. The Oxford meeting involved Parker, Holm and Ashcroft as contributors; the Maastricht meeting involved Agich, Widdershoven and Hurwitz; the Groningen meeting involved Verkerk, Campbell and Withers; and the London meeting involved Gillon and Savulescu. Initially, since the project had begun as a reaction to the predominance of principlist and utilitarian approaches to clinical ethics, the plan was to invite Raanan Gillon and Julian Savulescu to write responses to the other chapters, discussing how far their approaches could encompass or respond to the criticisms of their respective principlist and utilitarian approaches. In the course of preparing the book it became clear that this sort of 'contest' was inappropriate, and in a sense unfair to Raa and Julian (being put into a defensive role) and to everyone else (being made to engage in a conflict that many of them felt was no more than a difference in perspective). In a sense this was a little reaction to the very combative approach often found in bioethics, at least in theoretical work, where people take sides. Yet in clinical ethics, the aim is normally to avoid taking sides, to get participants to understand each other's viewpoints and to seek consensus or at least understanding. We feel that this was a valuable lesson. At each meeting Lucassen presented the case for the benefit of the contributors and guests, and this process of discussion led to some refinements of her text. All contributions were then collated and edited, at which point the present Introduction, and the two concluding chapters were prepared.

The order of the book is as follows. Anneke Lucassen's case report opens the main part of the book. Brian Hurwitz's chapter introduces the ideas of narrative analysis and narrative ethics. This approach concentrates on the way the case is reported, and examines how different ways of telling the story influence how we think about it, in particular how different ways personalities in the story represent their points of view shapes what happens and shapes what alternatives seem to be live possibilities. Developing some of the insights of narrative analysis, Alastair Campbell introduces the approach of virtue ethics. The link between narrative and virtue approaches is in the concept of character, from the narrative viewpoint, 'characters' are agents in the story and we are interested in how lifelike or rounded they are. But this also has a moral dimension, when one considers how lifelike or rounded we appear to ourselves or to others, and this is intimately connected to the idea of a virtuous individual and human flourishing, which is central in virtue ethics. Guy Widdershoven's chapter responds to this in his presentation of 'hermeneutic' ethics, which stresses the importance of developing a framework of understanding that can encompass all parties' different 'horizons of understanding' and hence stresses the importance of relationships as both sustaining and being sustained by the effort to understand.

Richard Ashcroft suggests that there are limits to understanding, and that both social structure and individual attempts to control their situation will always imply that power relationships can make relationships of regard and mutual recognition unstable. He explores whether there can be an ethic of power, suggesting that it lies in the effort to secure recognition of the vulnerability of each party. Rob Withers develops these ideas in his 'post-structuralist' reading of the case, focusing on the role of time and uncertainty in the case, to suggest that an ethic of vulnerability can be grounded in a different way to that suggested by Ashcroft. Withers' arguments about uncertainty apply to uncertainty about the motives of others and to one's own preferences, and as such mount a challenge to utilitarianism. Julian Savulescu responds by showing what a classical utilitarian approach can do, illustrating the difference between the vulgar utilitarianism frequently practised and what a more sophisticated form can actually do. Marian Verkerk develops an account of a feminist ethics-of-care approach to the case, which gives a feminist reading of the personal and power relationships, challenging the emphases on these given by Ashcroft. Michael Parker then describes a 'deliberative-ethics' approach that seeks to encompass both the formal requirements of fair discussion implied in the debate between Hurwitz, Widdershoven and Campbell, Withers, Ashcroft and Verkerk, and the substantive requirements of reason at stake in the debate between Withers, Ashcroft, Savulescu and Verkerk.

Raanan Gillon describes the classical principlist approach to case analysis, arguing that its strength lies in its ability to produce clear action-guiding recommendations, although, as he shows, this can require considerable subtlety and nuance. In common with the other authors he stresses the need for good ethical judgement in addition to the formal deduction of

conclusions from premises. George Agich, in his chapter on the phenomenological approach, suggests that the solution to the need for judgement may lie
in the way critical reason can uncover the constitutive assumptions that
underlie the experience of the case that each party has, and thus lead to a
reconception of what is at stake, which can produce a resolution. Finally,
Søren Holm indicates that a correct appreciation of the case may depend on
the need for reliable empirical information and suggests how case analysis can
become clarified through obtaining and reflecting on such information.

The book concludes with two looks back at the main part of the book: the
first is by the philosophers on the editorial team (Parker, Ashcroft, Verkerk
and Widdershoven), who draw out the similarities and differences between
the approaches described and assess the outcome of the 'philosophical
experiment' described above. Finally, Anneke Lucassen reflects on the process
of writing the book and engaging with philosophers from the perspective of a
working clinician.

REFERENCES

Beauchamp, T. and Childress, J. (2001). *Principles of Biomedical Ethics,* 5th edn.
     Oxford: Oxford University Press.
De Beauvoir, S. (1969). *A Very Easy Death.* London: Penguin.
Brody, H. (2003). *Stories of Sickness,* 2nd edn. Oxford: Oxford University Press.
Gilligan, C. (1993). *In a Different Voice: Psychological Theory and Women's
     Development.* Cambridge, Mass.: Harvard University Press.
Hunter, K. M. (1991). *Doctors' Stories: The Narrative Structure of Medical Knowledge.*
     Princeton, New Jersey: Princeton University Press.
Hursthouse, R. (1987). *Beginning Lives.* Oxford: Blackwell.
Jonsen, A. and Toulmin, S. (1988). *The Abuse of Casuistry.* London: University of
     California Press.
Sherwin, S. (1992). *No Longer Patient: Feminist Ethics and Health Care.* Philadelphia:
     Temple University Press.
Zaner, R. M. (1988). *Ethics and the Clinical Encounter.* Englewood Cliffs, New Jersey:
     Prentice Hall.

Families and genetic testing: the case of Jane and Phyllis

Anneke Lucassen

We share much of our genetic make-up with members of our biological family. This means that genetic information about one person is also sometimes, to a greater or lesser extent, information about that person's relatives. A genetic test can sometimes therefore diagnose or predict disease not only in the individual tested but also in his or her biological relatives.

The familial nature of the information produced by genetic tests raises questions about the legal and ethical obligations of healthcare professionals to disclose or withhold genetic information about patients to their at-risk relatives. Such questions are brought into sharp focus by clinical genetic situations in which different members of the same family are all 'patients' of one clinician but each attends the clinic independently with separate issues and agendas that need to be addressed. In such situations each patient is owed a duty of care by that clinician, who may feel pulled in different directions by the differing needs of the family members, and may feel unclear about how to prioritise each. Such questions are particularly difficult when family members are in conflict but they also arise when members have simply lost touch with each other. In such cases, there can be an ethical conflict between preserving the confidentiality of one patient on the one hand and the right of other family members to know information about their genetic status and risk of disease on the other.

Such problems are not new. The speciality of clinical genetics has always dealt with families, and with the tensions or lack of contact between family members. Different opinions within families are certainly not new. However, in the past, and until relatively recently, the only advice geneticists were able to provide consisted largely of estimates of risk of inheriting or transmitting a particular genetic condition. With the advent of genetic testing for an increasing number of conditions, it is now possible in some cases to infer or produce reasonably accurate information about actual inheritance.

In some cases, the ability of a genetic test to deliver useful prognostic or predictive information to an individual patient is dependent on the prior

Case Analysis in Clinical Ethics, ed. Richard Ashcroft, Anneke Lucassen, Michael Parker, Marian Verkerk, Guy Widdershoven. Published by Cambridge University Press.

identification of the causative genetic alteration in that particular family. This is usually only possible in a living family member who is actually affected by the condition. So this means that an unaffected member of a family who wants to know whether they have inherited a condition or a tendency towards a condition may need the co-operation of an affected relative in order to make an accurate test possible. This introduces another familial element into the practice of genetics.

In many families there is a willingness – and even an eagerness – to share genetic information of this kind, but in others conflict or separation results in situations where the clinician has to choose between preserving the confidentiality of one relative and making predictive genetic testing available to another. In such cases, where an accurate and useful test is only possible if the familial mutation has been identified, such conflicts can be difficult to resolve.

The following clinical case (see also Appendix I) highlights just such a conflict. The case, which is a construct composed from several cases I have encountered as a clinical geneticist, is also informed by a number of different stories told to me while seeing families clinically.

Jane's story

I have always known that most women in my family develop breast cancer, usually at a young age, and that they eventually die from it. I suppose when I was in my teens and twenties I knew it but it seemed remote to *me*. Once I reached my thirties and had my own two daughters things started to feel different. I worried more about developing cancer and about not being there for my girls. I worried that they too might have got our family curse. While my girls were little I always had other things to think about, but now that they're a bit older I think about it all the time.

The worries often loom large in the early hours when I lie awake fretting. My husband eventually persuaded me to see the doctor. He said I should go to see her because I didn't know what could be done these days and that treatments must be different from when mum and her mum developed cancer. At about the same time I also saw an article in the newspaper about genetic testing for women like me and I went to ask my GP about it. She was very good and gave me a lot of time. She talked a bit about mammograms and how to examine my own breasts. She didn't know much about genetic testing but said she'd refer me on to a specialist.

After several weeks of waiting I was sent a family history questionnaire to fill in. It asked about details of the cancers in my family, which hospitals my relatives had been treated at, how old they were and all sorts of other questions. I spent days filling it in. I found it hard and upsetting to complete.

After several months I finally got an appointment to see the specialist. She told me that it did sound like there was a rogue gene in my family that could explain all the cancers. She gave me lots of information, most of which I don't remember now, but I do remember her saying that there is a possibility that I may not have inherited the rogue gene. My mum had two copies of the gene and only one was faulty. When mum had us, she only passed on only one copy, either the normal one *or* the faulty one, so it was 'heads or tails' each time she had a child. If I didn't get it, I'm unlikely to get cancer young; if I did, then I probably will. The only problem is that we can't really tell whether I have or haven't got the relevant gene as the tests aren't yet very good. In order for me to have an accurate test, the researchers would first need to find the particular rogue gene in an affected person in my family since each family can have a slightly different type of rogue gene. For the test to be accurate in me, they need to know exactly which gene fault they are looking for before they test me for it. If they tested me without this first bit of information, and I tested negative, it could mean that I hadn't got mum's rogue gene but, and this was the big but, it could also mean that I had got it but the researchers had not been able to find it because their tests aren't good enough to pick up all the different types of gene faults.

If they knew what to look for, they'd be able to offer me a straight 'yes' or 'no' answer; but if they don't, a test isn't really going to help me to decide not to have an operation. Since all the women in my family seem to die from cancer rather quickly there is no-one who is affected that I can ask to undertake this first stage test. Without this, testing me seems like a bit of a 'don't know' test.[1]

At the end of the meeting, the doctor said it might help if I got some more information about mum's relations. I think that Great Uncle Stan emigrated to Australia in the 1970s and the doctor said finding out if maybe he had had any daughters with breast cancer who were still alive could be helpful. I know very little about mum's family really as I was only 21 when she died. I was her baby and I think she didn't want to tell me things that she thought might upset me. I did know Auntie Phyllis was still alive although I hadn't seen her since mum died.

When I asked him, Uncle George told me Phyllis still lived in the same house, but when I finally got in touch with her she didn't really have any more information. She's a rather grumpy thing. She and mum had some row over money and she went on about mum being the spoilt one. I found the visit rather depressing. She looked old and not very well but she's only in her 50s.

By the time I went for my second appointment at the genetics clinic I'd done loads of reading around the subject and talked to a woman who ran a support group who had a very similar story to mine. She had had an operation called a prophylactic mastectomy, which removes almost all of your breasts so that you can't develop cancer in them. The genetics doctor said that there was evidence to show that women like me who had this operation probably did better than women who just examined themselves and had mammograms. To be honest, I was already pretty convinced this was the way to go before that, especially as my husband also thought this was a good idea, but also because genetic testing in me probably wasn't really going to be that helpful for a few years yet. I just thought, if I have the operation then I can stop worrying. I was so fed up of having this gnawing anxiety constantly in the back of my head.

Phyllis's story

I knew I was doing pretty well to get to 50 without developing cancer, all the other women in the family had got it much before that, but when I felt the lump in my breast I knew straight away that it was cancer.

Everything moved very quickly – before I knew it I'd had the operation and I was told I was 'doing very well'. The oncology doctor looking after me was young and very energetic. He said that because I had so many relatives with cancer that the cancer might be due to something I'd inherited. He said a blood test might show this. If it did show it then he would probably suggest a different treatment than if it didn't. I don't think he ever asked whether I wanted the test, he just took the blood sample. About a year later when I'd clean forgotten all about it, I got a letter from him saying that the test had found something and that he'd send me on to some genetic people to talk about it. To be honest I found the genetic people were rather wishy-washy. They never seemed to have a clear 'yes' or 'no' answer to my questions. They said the result was a faulty gene, but that there wasn't good enough evidence to show that it should alter my treatment in any way, especially as I was now well. They were more interested in my relations who hadn't got cancer, which was a bit of a cheek. I told the doctor how I'd nursed my mother and my sister when they were dying. Neither of them thanked me for it. My sister and I had a huge row about money just before she died – it was dreadful. I wasn't even mentioned in her will and the family completely ignored me afterwards. I don't feel I owe them anything. So no, I wasn't happy with them letting others know of my test result. I'm not in touch with them. It is my result, not anyone else's business. I'm fed up with being blamed for anything that goes wrong in our family.

The general practitioner's story

I first realised there was a problem when I got the letter from the clinical geneticist. Phyllis wasn't happy to divulge the result of genetic testing to her family members, but in theory the result could be used by her niece, Jane, to decide whether to have a prophylactic mastectomy or not. Without the result Jane might have the operation unnecessarily, i.e. undergo it when in fact she hadn't inherited the cancer trait.

Of course, it wouldn't have been so much of an issue for us had not both of the two women been registered at our practice. My partner looks after Phyllis, and I had met Jane on several occasions. We discussed it at a practice meeting. My partner felt very strongly, and I think I agree with him, that neither we nor anyone else, should break Phyllis's confidentiality. She specifically said that she does not want anyone to know. I think her main reasons are that she would feel blamed by the family and I think that is reasonable.

General Medical Council guidelines say we should only break confidentiality in a very serious or life-threatening condition. From what I understand, there is not enough evidence to show clearly that prophylactic bilateral mastectomies in Jane will reduce her chance of dying from breast cancer. Plus, it's a major and mutilating piece of surgery. I think she should just have regular screens. My partner wondered why they couldn't just test Jane for the gene fault that they've found in Phyllis but without letting Phyllis know. I thought that was probably a good way round. However, when I spoke to the genetics team they indicated they had already explained to Jane – before they knew she and Phyllis were related – that genetic testing wasn't going to be helpful without first having obtained the results of this same test on an affected family member. Going back to Jane and changing that story would mean she'd be able to infer things about Phyllis's state of health.

The oncologist's story

I attended a one-day seminar on advances in genetics and oncology a few months before I first saw Phyllis, and this suggested that the treatment of hereditary breast and ovarian cancer should be more aggressive than that of sporadic cancer. I had this in mind when I sent off for the BRCA genetic test on Phyllis (see Appendix II). She had consented to lots of investigative blood tests as part of her diagnosis and treatment. I did not specifically discuss with her the consequences of a genetic-test result for her family but that was not my prime reason for performing the test – I wanted clarification on the nature of her cancer. I have discussed the case with the clinical genetics department and I now realise the genetic-test result has created difficulties. Partly this is because of the low sensitivity of current testing, which is the ability of a test correctly to screen gene-free individuals as negative. Sensitivity is likely to improve in the future and when it does we will no longer be dependent on results in one relative in order to undertake a test of adequate specificity in another but it may of course be that similar dilemmas will continue to arise in other genetic tests.

I can see that a genetic test is unusual because it can reveal information about people other than those who actually have the test. Nevertheless, ultimately I am responsible for the patient in front of me and if I have evidence to suggest that my treatment of a cancer might be different depending on the result of a genetic test then I think it appropriate to do that test without having to seek the consent of other relatives who might also have an interest in the result of that test. I do think it is appropriate for the geneticists or counsellors to try to facilitate discussion between the two women. But at the end of the day we shouldn't have to consider the effects of a test on all family members before proceeding with it, that's just not practical or feasible.

The geneticist's story

Jane attended the genetics clinic asking for a genetic test to see whether she'd inherited her family trait for breast cancer. She'd read about genetic testing in a magazine, but unfortunately the magazine had not spelt out the current limitations of such testing. I told her that *at present* genetic testing for breast cancer susceptibility is a two-stage process. In order for her to have a test that tells her whether or not she has inherited a familial trait for breast cancer (a *predictive* test) a first-stage test must be done on an *affected* family member which will then enable a subsequent test on Jane herself to provide a definitive yes/no answer (a *diagnostic* test).

Without a predictive test on an affected family member with breast cancer that would be able to identify a causative or pathogenic mutation, a diagnostic test on Jane would have a very low sensitivity. This is because there are at least two and probably more different genes that, if mutated, cause a high risk of breast cancer. Hundreds of different mutations in these genes in different families have been described. Current technologies can at best pick up 70–80% of these mutations and in fact most testing in this country detects a smaller percentage. This means that testing Jane directly is unlikely to help her decide against a prophylactic mastectomy: a negative test would not usefully distinguish between whether the mutation was not present (that she has not inherited it) or whether it had simply not been identified due to the limitations of current techniques. So a 'negative' result could not reliably be taken to mean she had a reduced chance of having inherited the cancer trait. However, a negative predictive test, if the diagnostic test had already shown up the relevant mutation in Jane's family, could accurately tell her that her risk of breast cancer is now roughly the same as that in the general population. Although this risk is roughly equal to a 1 in 10 chance in a woman's lifetime, sporadic cancers are usually late-onset and Jane could therefore be reassured that her chances of developing young-onset cancers seen in her family were extremely low, and we would advise against prophylactic surgery. *Predictive* testing, as the magazine suggested, can be highly accurate, but it is not informative if we don't know which particular mutation we're looking for, and for that we need to find the mutation in an affected relative.

When I first met Jane she told me that all her relatives who had had cancer were long since dead. Only later were we referred Phyllis, together with her BRCA1 mutation result. This doesn't happen that often, as we usually initiate testing, but there are a few keen oncologists around who feel they might as well send the test off if there is a strong family history. When this has happened before there hasn't usually been an issue about disclosing the result to other family members since that is usually the main motivation for doing the test. However, it is clear that the test result does also have implications for Phyllis. It now gives her a clearer risk of ovarian cancer (up to a 60% chance in her lifetime) and she may want to consider a prophylactic oophorectomy to reduce her risk. If and when there is good evidence to suggest that the treatment of gene-mutation-related cancers is different from that of sporadic cancers, then I guess this situation will happen more often.

Usually, in cases where the *diagnostic* test has revealed a pathogenic mutation, we'd leave the onus up to the person we see to contact their relatives and inform them of the possibility of a *predictive* test. We feel we cannot directly approach people who have not been referred to us. Of course we have no idea how often such subsequent communication simply never takes place, leaving people with a large degree of uncertainty, or even ignorance, about whether or not they will develop young-onset breast cancer, which could, in theory, be removed by a predictive genetic test. But we also do not know how many women in this situation would want to know the genetic nature of the condition in an affected family.

In this case, however, the two women were referred to us independently and were both patients of the regional genetics service. I saw Jane and my colleague saw Phyllis. It was not until a case conference that we realised the two were related. By that time I'd spelt out the problems of genetic testing to Jane which included an explanation of the fact that she couldn't have a useful predictive test unless we could first find the pathogenic mutation in an affected relative. She'd even sought Phyllis out and spoken to her but Phyllis hadn't told her about her cancer or her test result. We couldn't therefore fudge the issue with Jane. She's an intelligent woman; if we'd suddenly said 'Oh we can do a test after all' – and just looked for the mutation that we knew to be present in Phyllis – then Jane would have realised that we must have information from one of her relatives and she'd probably have been straight round to Phyllis.

I can see that it would be breaking Phyllis's confidentiality to tell Jane. It's true that there is not yet any research evidence that clearly shows that women who are likely to have one of these dominant breast-cancer genes should have prophylactic bilateral mastectomies recommended to them. But there *is* accumulating evidence that the lifetime risk of cancer following such an operation is significantly reduced; short-term follow-up studies of these women have shown that the cancer incidence is much lower in these women than in the same-risk women who are just screened regularly. However, there are not yet any data that suggest the *mortality* from breast cancer is reduced if these women have such an operation. Such data may never be collected, partly because the number of families are small and partly because randomisation of studies might be difficult; anecdotally, women may either want or not want such a major operation based more on their family's experience rather than on a risk figure that we provide for them.

When women have seen many members of their family die from breast cancer, I think it not unreasonable to discuss such an operation as there is enough evidence to suggest it is *likely* to be of benefit. If there was absolutely clear evidence of benefit then I would find it easier to argue that breaking Phyllis's confidentiality is justified in order to prevent serious harm, i.e. an unnecessary major operation. Since we do not direct women to have such an operation when we clearly know they have a gene mutation (but only suggest it as an option) can we say that breaking confidentiality is justified in this case? Or should we advise Jane that there is not enough evidence for surgery in *any* case? Even without these ambiguities I feel it is difficult to know how to proceed when there is such a direct clash of interests between family members. Clearly, negotiation might help but my colleague has tried hard to suggest to Phyllis that it would be in the interest of her family to disclose (and that in itself is difficult to do without breaking Jane's confidentiality), but she just doesn't see it as in her best interest. Phyllis feels she would be blamed and stigmatised. She's a sad and isolated woman who shouldn't be bullied into doing something she thinks will bring her harm.

Jane is pretty much decided on having prophylactic mastectomies, yet there is a 50% chance this will be unnecessary. This is, however, a situation she is only prepared to tolerate because she thinks there is no way of getting a more accurate risk figure. But we know this is not the case. How would she feel if in years to come she found out that she had never needed the operation and that we had had the information available at the time to show this yet we allowed her to proceed with major surgery regardless? I feel that in these situations, Phyllis's test result really belongs to her whole family, not just to her. She has information that is highly relevant to Jane, yet she is withholding it. I think that we should make it a condition of testing in the first place, that it will be all right to use the test result for the benefit of other family members. Of course, I realise this may prevent people like Phyllis taking the test in the first place, so Jane would be no better off, but at least we wouldn't be in the difficult dilemma we are in now. Personally, I feel it is wrong to be referring Jane on for such major surgery when I have information, which I cannot share with her, that may make this surgery unnecessary. We've tried our hardest to negotiate with Phyllis and to persuade her of the potential benefit to unaffected relatives but it seems to fall on deaf ears. I don't know which side of the fence I'd come down on if Jane was not contemplating major surgery, if she just wanted to know in order to be more certain of her risks, but I feel the potential surgery shifts the balance. I think Jane should be told about Phyllis's result, and Phyllis about the disclosure, in as sensitive a way possible.

Author's comment

While this case is a composite of many different cases, I hope it serves to highlight the sort of dilemmas that are faced by professionals looking after both families and individuals. The discussion is centred around breast cancer and ways of detecting or preventing it. Jane is potentially also at risk of ovarian cancer. The lifetime risks for this cancer in someone who has inherited a BRCA1 mutation is up to 60%. Screening is of unproven benefit although research studies on this are ongoing. Because of the lack of effective screening for ovarian cancer, some women consider prophylactic removal of the ovaries to be the right course to take, and this may well be an attractive option for Jane as she has already completed her family. Although not such a major operation as a mastectomy, at Jane's age she might need a period of hormone-replacement therapy to prevent osteoporosis. Again, her options would be much clearer if a predictive test were possible for her. This additional risk of ovarian cancer adds yet further complexities to the case: what role should requests for additional major surgery such as bilateral oophorectomy play in weighing up whether to disclose or not? If Jane were not contemplating any surgery but wanted to continue with screening instead would that make a difference to whether Phyllis's result should be disclosed? In this case, Jane might still be availing herself of unevaluated and expensive screening for many years that could be shown to be unnecessary if Phyllis's result was disclosed.

A criticism of the particular case I have chosen might be that it presents a dilemma only because of the technicalities of a genetic test in its infancy. Once genetic testing is more advanced, testing of an individual will be less dependent on initial testing of another relative. This of course may turn out to be true, but testing for other conditions may become available and also have to go through the same uncertain stages. Moreover, even when routine testing of everyone's entire genome is possible there will be many other possible scenarios in which information on one person, if not disclosed to a relative, may prevent that relative knowing their risk. These include the following scenarios:

A woman with a young disabled son finds out that his problems are due to muscular dystrophy. She is a carrier of the condition. Her sister has a 50% chance, therefore, that she is also a carrier and has just revealed she is 10 weeks pregnant but concerned about bringing a disabled child into the world. The woman refuses to tell her sister of the risk as she thinks she may terminate a pregnancy. She herself is opposed to termination. Routine testing for muscular dystrophy would not be available in pregnancy unless a specific familial mutation were known. (Parker and Lucassen 2004)

A man with a family history of Huntington's disease (HD) who has tested positive, marries a woman who wants to start a family. He does not tell her of his diagnosis as he is worried that she will leave him. (Lucassen and Parker 2004)

Many other conditions exist where confirmation of what the actual condition in an affected relative is, is of importance for the accuracy of the test in their relatives, e.g. family history of suspected HD again, in which there may be a need to confirm that the dementing illness in the relative is in fact HD, rather than another dementing illness, before a predictive test is accurate.

It might also be suggested, as a criticism of the case, that, had the time sequence of this case been different the dilemma might have disappeared. Had Phyllis been referred to clinical genetics *before* genetic testing had been carried out, for example, consent could have been asked of her at this point to disclose any result to her relatives if it were likely to prove helpful to them. This could even have been made a precondition to testing. Some genetic departments are now doing this as part of their consent process but it is not known how many people are thereby deterred from testing altogether, or indeed how many would refuse to accept the conditions to consent. If people are deterred, then clearly Jane's position is no better than in the case as described (because the test would not have been carried out), but at least then the clinicians would not be faced with the dilemma of knowing information that could help Jane but not be able to disclose it. The placing of conditions such as these on patients' access to genetic testing raises a number of important ethical issues in its own right of course. Could it ever be ethical to deny a patient access to a test unless he or she were willing to consent to the use of its results for family members?

The case might also have been different if Jane were referred after the team already knew of Phyllis's existence and both of her relationship with Jane and her wish for non-disclosure. Under these circumstances, it might have been possible to fudge the issue in discussion with Jane. If the geneticist hadn't explained the current limitations of testing so thoroughly it would have been possible simply to test Jane for Phyllis's mutation without anyone knowing and then give her a result. Even so, this would not, of course, constitute informed consent and fudging of this type could easily come to light at a later stage leaving professional probity open to question.

This is an area that requires much greater public and professional discussion and debate and I hope that the chapters in this book will contribute to and enlighten such debate.

NOTE

1 For more information about inherited breast cancer and genetic testing see also patient information leaflet in Appendix II.

REFERENCES

Lucassen, A. and Parker, M. (2004). Confidentiality and 'serious harm' in genetics: preserving the confidentiality of one patient and preventing harms to relatives. *Eur J Human Gen*, **12**(2), 93–7.

Parker, M. and Lucassen, A. (2004). Genetic information: a joint account? *BMJ*, **329**, 165–7.

APPENDIX I Family diagram

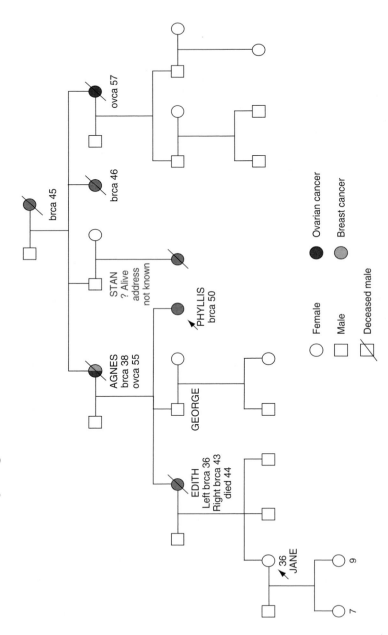

APPENDIX II Patient information leaflet

This leaflet has been produced by Anneke Lucassen for the Wessex Clinical Genetics Service, Southampton, UK.

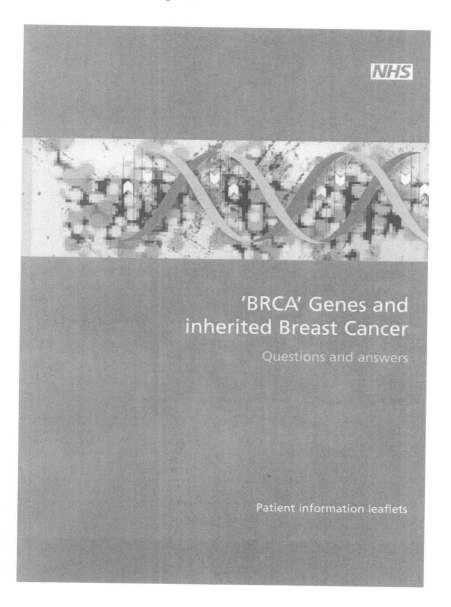

NHS

'BRCA' Genes and inherited Breast Cancer

Questions and answers

Patient information leaflets

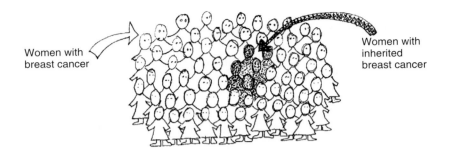

Women with breast cancer

Women with inherited breast cancer

This booklet has been written for people who have a family history of breast and/or ovarian cancer which could be explained by an inherited factor. It aims to answer some of the questions you may have.

Is breast cancer inherited?

Usually not. In only about 5 to 10 of every hundred women with breast cancer is the cancer thought to be due to a strong inherited factor. This factor is an alteration (called a mutation) in a gene inherited from a parent. Two genes have been identified that cause a large increase in the risk of developing breast cancer when they are altered. They are called BRCA1 and BRCA2 (Breast cancer gene 1 and 2).

What is BRCA1 and BRCA2?

BRCA1 and 2 are genes that everybody has which make a protein that is important for the normal function of cells. A mutation in these genes alters the message the genes send to the body, which increases the chances of developing breast and/or ovarian cancer.

How are BRCA genes inherited?

We all have two copies of each of our genes; one we get from our mother, the other from our father. When we have children we randomly pass on just one of each of our pairs of genes. If a person has a mutation in one of a pair of genes, each of his or her children has a 50:50 chance of inheriting it or not. The mutation can be inherited from either parent, although the chances of a man developing breast cancer are much lower than for a woman.

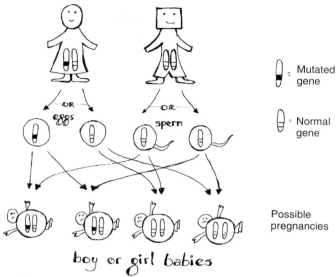

: Mutated gene

: Normal gene

Possible pregnancies

boy or girl babies

This shows a mother with a faulty gene but it could be either partner
For every child there is a 50%, or 1 in 2, chance of inheriting the mutation

**If a person has not inherited BRCA mutation then they cannot
pass it on to their children.**

How do I know if the cancer in my family is due to a mutation in a BRCA gene?

If you have several closely related family members (such as sisters, mother, grandmother, aunts who are blood relatives) with breast and/or ovarian cancer, and if their cancers occurred at a young age (usually below the age of 50), there may be a breast cancer (BRCA) gene mutation in your family. Remember that even if this is the case, you may not have inherited it (see above).

Can I have a test to see if the breast cancer in my family is due to a mutation in a BRCA gene?

This may be possible. A person's genes can be examined from a blood sample. However, because only a small proportion of people with breast cancer will have a BRCA mutation, and the test is technically difficult and takes a long time, it is at present only offered to people with a very strong family history of breast/ovarian cancer at a young age. Without this sort of family story, the test is unlikely to show any mutations.

I have got a very strong family history, how do I go about testing?

We need to start by obtaining a sample of blood from a relative in your family who has had breast or ovarian cancer and look for a mutation. Different families with breast/ovarian cancer have different mutations in the BRCA1 or 2 genes or even other genes that have yet to be discovered. We need to find which, if any, is the mutation for your family. Genetic testing is currently technically difficult and therefore a lengthy process. We know that at present we cannot find all the different mutations. Our techniques are constantly improving and in years to come testing will be more straightforward but at present there will be many families who have a gene mutation that the laboratory cannot yet find.

What if a relative with breast or ovarian cancer is not available? Can I be tested even if I have never had cancer?

The test is very difficult to interpret without knowing if a mutation exists in the family and which one it is. One of the reasons for this is that if we test a person who has not had cancer and the test does not find a mutation, we cannot tell whether that is good news (and you have not inherited the mutation), or whether the test has not been able to find a mutation that is in fact present (because of the current technical limitations of the test).

Testing you without knowing the mutation for your family would mean we could not reassure you that you had not inherited the cancer tendency. In reality in a family with one of the BRCA1 or 2 mutations which cause cancer, there is always a 50% (1 in 2) chance of this (see diagram).

So testing is a two-stage process?

Yes. The first step, the **"diagnostic test"** looks for the mutation in an affected relative. If we cannot find it, then at present testing is not possible in you. We would hope that testing will improve and that a mutation will be found in the future.

If we do find the mutation in an affected relative then we can examine your blood to see whether or not you have the same mutation. This is called a **"predictive test"**. This second test is very accurate and takes just a few weeks. There is a 50% chance it will be positive (you have inherited) and a 50% chance it will be negative (you have not inherited the gene mutation). A predictive test in the presence of a known mutation in a family member is highly accurate.

Does everyone who inherits a mutation in a BRCA gene get breast or ovarian cancer?

No. The risk of developing these cancers is high, but not 100%. We do not yet know why some women with the mutation develop cancer and some do not. Lifestyle or other genetic factors may play a role.

Remember that the risk of developing cancer is not the same as the risk of dying from cancer. Even if cancer develops, there is a chance that the disease can be cured if detected and treated early.

How high is my risk of cancer if I have inherited a BRCA mutation?

The risk of developing breast cancer in your lifetime may be as high as 80% and as high as 60% for ovarian cancer. That is, up to 8 out of every 10 women with the BRCA mutation will develop breast cancer at some point in their lives; up to 6 out of every 10 women with the mutation will develop ovarian cancer. The exact risk varies depending on where in the gene the mutation lies and on possibly other genetic and lifestyle factors.

If I have not inherited a BRCA mutation can I still get cancer?

Unfortunately, yes. Although the risk is then no higher than for anyone else in the general population, there is still a chance of developing cancer, because cancer can occur for other reasons. Every woman has a roughly 10% (1 in 10) chance of developing breast cancer in their lifetime, so even with a negative gene test, there is still a chance of developing breast cancer. However, this cancer is more likely to develop at a later age than a cancer due to a BRCA gene mutation.

What happens if a man has a mutation in a BRCA gene?

Men do not have as high a risk of developing breast cancer as women do, but they can get breast cancer. There may also be a slightly increased risk of developing prostate cancer. The exact increase in risk is not yet known. Research studies are looking at this.

Men can pass on the mutation to their sons and daughters.

Are BRCA1/2 the only genes that can cause hereditary breast cancer?

No. Probably about three-quarters of all inherited breast cancer is due to mutations in BRCA1 or BRCA2. There are likely to be other genes that increase the risk of developing breast cancer which have not yet been found.

If I have a BRCA mutation when will I develop cancer?

You may never develop cancer at all. It is not possible to predict whether you will or will not develop cancer or at what age you will develop it.

What can be done about the risk of developing breast or ovarian cancer?

- Some women will want to be followed closely by their doctor to detect cancer as early as possible, since treatment is more effective in the early stages. This may include regular **breast examinations** and **mammograms**. Unfortunately these tests will not be able to pick up all cancers. In general, mammograms are more able to pick up cancers in older women. In younger women the doctors need to plan carefully how often mammograms are done because they carry a greater risk. The benefits of mammography are not entirely clear in younger women.
- Some women might consider preventative or **prophylactic surgery** (removing the breasts or ovaries before cancer occurs). This does not completely eliminate the chance of cancer but will reduce it by a large amount. Other leaflets describe this in more detail.
- There are studies underway on different types of **drugs** that may decrease the risk of developing these cancers.

These can all be discussed in more detail at the clinic.

What is the advantage of predictive BRCA testing?

Women who have a mutation in a BRCA gene are at high risk of developing breast and ovarian cancer. Knowing your risks may help you with decisions about your life and may allow you to take action to reduce your risks. You can talk to your doctor about the screening and other options available to you. However, it is important to know that at present there is no method of detection or prevention that has been proven to be completely effective. Despite this, some women would rather know whether they have inherited a BRCA mutation than live with the uncertainty.

Remember there is a 50% chance that the test will show you have not inherited the mutation. This means you cannot have passed it on to any of your children or future children. You will also not need any screening until you start the population screening at 50 years.

Remember "predictive" means a test on a person who has not had cancer but who is closely related to someone who has and in whom a mutation has been found.

What are the risks of BRCA testing?

If a mutation is found that increases your risk of developing cancer it may affect your ability to get **insurance** (e.g. health, life, disability). Currently the insurance industry has agreed it will not ask about genetic testing for the majority of policies, but this position may change in the future.

You may want to review your insurance before testing. You should talk to your doctor about how the information will be kept in your medical records.

Some people experience many emotions when they are told they have a gene that increases their risk of cancer. Anger, shock, anxiety, worry about their health, worry or guilt about possibly passing the gene on to children are all normal reactions. Some people may also feel guilty if they do not carry the change in the gene when other close family members do so.

Remember that we can tell you your risk is increased but we cannot tell you for certain when or even if you will develop cancer.

Genetic testing in a family can affect other family members, they may need to be told that they too are at increased risk or unexpected information may be revealed, for example, someone may disclose that a family member is adopted. Therefore, genetic testing may sometimes affect relationships within families.

Is there an alternative to genetic testing?

You may choose not to have genetic testing. Whether or not you are tested, you should talk to your doctor about starting a programme to detect cancer early.

I've heard of research studies involving people with a family history of cancer. How can I find out more?

There are currently several different national and international research studies. More information can be obtained from the address overleaf. It is important to remember that research studies may not benefit you directly, but may help others or future generations.

Talk to your doctor about all of the options before deciding on a plan of action that is best for you.

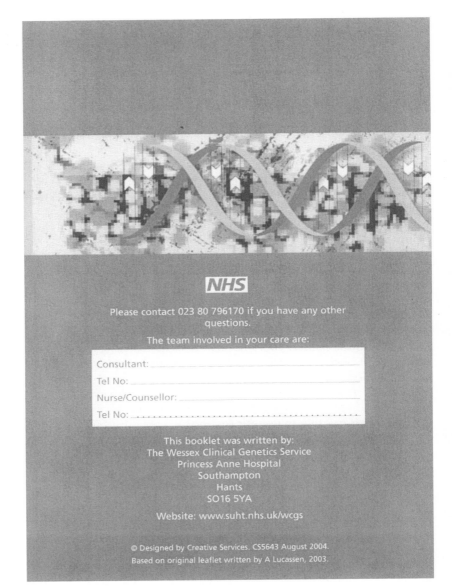

Please contact 023 80 796170 if you have any other
questions.

The team involved in your care are:

Consultant: _____

Tel No: _____

Nurse/Counsellor: _____

Tel No: _____

This booklet was written by:
The Wessex Clinical Genetics Service
Princess Anne Hospital
Southampton
Hants
SO16 5YA

Website: www.suht.nhs.uk/wcgs

© Designed by Creative Services. CS5643 August 2004.
Based on original leaflet written by A Lucassen, 2003.

3

Family access to shared genetic information: an analysis of the narrative

Brian Hurwitz

Narratives are the discursive form in which issues in medical ethics are apprehended, and communicated. What stories do 'is to narrate the life in time' (Forster 1971), not just in novels, but also in fact. Narrative discourse – 'someone telling someone else that something happened' (Smith 1981) – is an archetypal means of relating and reporting what is going on, one which also patterns understanding of events.

Many stories turn on conflicts of value, clashes of principle and the promise of resolution. Literature, understood broadly to include novels, biography, memoirs and journalistic accounts, offers readers and professional ethicists alike, potentially rich representations of situations finely graduated by moral viewpoint, ambiguity and complexity (Widdershoven and Smits 1996, Widdershoven and Sohl 1999). Literature can also depict and explore moral doubts and reasoning, and subject argument, motive and character to the scrutiny of a wide readership. In these ways stories both embody and structure our encounters with notions of 'right' and 'wrong' (MacIntyre 1981: 201, Guroian 1998).

Some narrative scholars argue that 'the most interesting parts of the moral world have to be 'read', rendered, construed, glossed, elucidated, and not merely described' (Walzer 1987) and find that novelists have more to teach them than philosophers about how to grapple with moral complexities (Booth 2002). Comprehending the moral content of stories involves making sense of feelings, thoughts and behaviour which engage narrative skills, knowledge of the fine grain of medical case histories and some fluency in philosophical analysis too (Levine 1998: 43). 'We are rational as well as affective beings' writes Edmund Pellegrino, and 'we respond to the story's moral arguments as well as the feelings it inspires. But to do this, not only must we enter the story but we must transcend it. Judging whether a story is good or bad is not just a literary judgement. Ethics subjects the story to a meta-narrative analysis. Reason and feeling, *logos* and *patheia*, are inextricable from the healing relationship and from ethical reflection' (Pellegrino 1997: 15).

Case Analysis in Clinical Ethics, ed. Richard Ashcroft, Anneke Lucassen, Michael Parker, Marian Verkerk, Guy Widdershoven. Published by Cambridge University Press.
© Cambridge University Press 2005.

In supplying 'detail, contextuality, complexity and appreciation of values' literature conjures up encounters with many hypothetical people who can summon sympathy and provoke introspection in readers (Levine 1998). Drama, in particular, engenders tragedy, awareness of situations – true dilemmas – in which no choice is a good choice, in which anxious consider-ations about free will and constraints imposed by circumstances, are forced upon an audience. In *After Virtue*, MacIntyre finds in the stage a metaphor well suited to discussion of the tragic and narrative dimensions of everyday life: 'We enter upon a stage which we did not design and we find ourselves part of an action that was not of our making. Each of us being a main character in his own drama, plays subordinate parts in the dramas of others, and each drama constrains the others . . . We are never more (and sometimes less) than the co-authors of our own narratives. Only in fantasy do we live what story we please' (MacIntyre 1981: 213).

The tools that narrative appreciation brings to moral discernment are those that promote the close reading of texts. They include analysis of story structure and style, and consideration of the effect of the narrator in orches-trating (controlling and conveying) information, and in eliciting or suppres-sing moral and personal viewpoints. Questions such as which elements in a story are given prominence and which remain behind the scenes or are omitted altogether, how convincing is a person's reasoning and how credible their behaviour may point to narrative gaps, embedded viewpoints, or bias in the way an ethics case is constructed. Focus on specific narrative devices, such as time passing, plot and depiction of character – devices employed not only by ethicists but also by historians, lawyers and clinicians – can bring to the fore interrelations between context and causality in case histories (Cobley 2001, Chambers 1994).

Tod Chambers argues for the absence of privileged and innocent composi-tions and readings of medical ethical problems. What is required for analysis of ethics cases, he urges, is a sophisticated response to the story on the part of readers and listeners, one that enables detailed attention to be paid to the 'constructedness' of ethical cases. Chambers shows how ethics reports are rhetorically framed so as to 'make readers see another's way of seeing as natural and self-evident' when it may not be (Chambers 1999), and he notes how commonly ethics case histories are composed in a depersonalised, 'naturalistic' style typical of the medical 'literature of fact', namely, the clinical case history (Chambers 2002).

Interestingly, the case of Jane and Phyllis is not typical of a clinical case history. Their case takes the form of a sequential survey of first-person accounts, which shifts the reader's attention from one character to another and from one detail to another seen from the differing per-spectives of individuals who both narrate and feature in the case. The reader is invited to respond to a mosaic of reflective viewpoints and moral positions, but can do so only after piecing together the individual accounts into a coherent narrative (Uspensky 1973: 60). The narrative reading of the care of Jane and Phyllis offered here gives weight, as Pellegrino calls for, to the reasoning, feeling and ethical components of the case (Pellegrino 1997: 15).

Piecing the jigsaw puzzle together

Each viewpoint in this case is presented as a first-person monologue. Jane begins her account portentously, addressing her remarks about 'the family curse' directly to the reader: 'I have always known that women in my family develop breast cancer, usually at an early age, and that they die from it.' Initially, her mood seems resigned and fateful, and the occasion somewhat confessional, which it is not. The impression gained is of inner speech and uncensored thoughts, which are made available to the reader. It is from the privacy of this inner, mental space that Jane tells her story, describing a family lineage in which breast cancer has appeared frequently over several generations, and has caused much suffering and premature death.

Early in her account, we are introduced to Jane's gathering sense of impending danger, both to herself and, by extension, to her daughters. However, if Jane's mood starts out as apparently one of resignation, it soon becomes clear, as her story unfolds, that a lively energy animates her determination to understand her situation. Something of Jane's complexity and roundedness of character is conveyed by the depiction of her as a person whose mood evolves. The case reveals Jane to be networked into family and social structures that provide her with information that supports development of her thoughts and attitudes. By contrast, these dynamic and individuating characteristics are less apparent in respect of the depiction of Phyllis.

Until recently, Jane tells us, she has been able to contain her anxiety at the prospect of developing breast cancer, but worry has now got the better of her. She has become anxious about what would happen to her daughters were she to contract breast cancer. Jane raises her concerns with her GP, i.e. her primary-care physician, who refers her to a clinical geneticist, and at this point Jane shares with readers a quite sophisticated understanding of the risk she believes she runs of developing breast cancer.[1] This understanding explains Jane's decision to contact Phyllis, the surviving sister of her mother (Edith), and the only family member whom Jane believes could provide her with the information she needs. However, she finds Phyllis unforthcoming.

What does Jane really think?

On meeting Phyllis, Jane perceives that Phyllis looks unwell and puts Phyllis's lack of interest in meeting up (after 15 years' estrangement) down to Phyllis's longstanding jealousy of Jane's mother, Edith, 'the spoilt one', and to family rows about money (which Jane clearly believes still rankle with Phyllis). Jane attributes Phyllis's unhelpfulness to an aspect of what she takes to be Phyllis's personality, namely her grumpiness.

How much of this case history, as it has unfolded so far, can we take at face value? Gilbert Ryle dubbed morally neutral descriptions of events and actions 'ethically thin'. The contraction of an eyelid, for example, may merely be an involuntary response to dust in the air, or it may seal a contract when a bidder throws a wink to an auctioneer, or be the conspiratorial wink that signals to a confederate to pull the trigger on an innocent victim. The meaning discerned in descriptions of events, Ryle argued, depends critically on the context supplied. In the same way that narrative contexts can transform the twitch of a muscle into an action associated with motives and desires, so narratives – by infusing what happens with meaningful relations – can 'thicken' our moral knowledge and understanding of events.

'She's rather a grumpy thing' is how Jane assesses Phyllis, a 'thin' description we realise. For to jump briefly to how Phyllis 'thickly' describes her own attitude and feeling towards her relations, Phyllis says 'I don't feel I owe them anything. So no, I wasn't happy with . . . letting others know of my test result. It was my result, not anyone else's business.'

Phyllis claims that her health information 'belongs' to Phyllis herself, and she wishes to control who is privy to it (Hurwitz 2002). She also hints that there could be circumstances, such as repayment of a debt, in which she would be prepared to divulge this information to others. But in Phyllis's view she bears no such debt to Jane, nor (for that matter) to anyone else in the family. From snippets of information elsewhere in the case history, it is clear that Phyllis actually holds the reverse to be true: Phyllis believes she is the person who is owed thanks, for all the care she provided to Edith, Jane's mother, when Edith was suffering from breast cancer. In Phyllis's view, no such gratitude has ever been forthcoming from Edith's family. On the contrary, Phyllis has been cut out of Edith's will and cut off from Edith's family.

Jane and Phyllis's meeting

Phyllis, at this stage, appears to have no empathic feelings towards Jane or her plight, and Jane seems to have no intimation of Phyllis's hurt, her real situation (one of suffering breast cancer alone) or of what motivates Phyllis's behaviour towards her. But what does Phyllis actually *know* of Jane's situation? Jane comes to see Phyllis for the first time since her mother died some 15 years ago, and what passes between them during this meeting is not at all clear from Jane's account. The case presented exquisitely highlights a failure of interpersonal exchange between Jane and Phyllis, a failure with roots in a longstanding constellation of family feelings and attitudes.

How convinced are we that Jane is really unaware that Phyllis has breast cancer? Jane is very likely to suspect precisely this fact, in view of Phyllis's position within the family lineage, and in view of Jane's own observation that Phyllis looks unwell. Is not the likelihood that Phyllis already has breast cancer a central part of Jane's very rationale for contacting Phyllis in the first place?

In this tale, Jane appears to be the sort of person who thinks through situations; there would have been little or no point in Jane seeking information from a family member who was *not* clearly at risk of developing (who possibly already has developed) breast cancer. The credibility of this reading of Jane's thinking can be confirmed in the text itself, by referring to Jane's clinical geneticist, who reveals that she feels unable to suggest a new (and false) factual basis for testing Jane genetically – by 'fudging the issue' of how this could be done without prior identification of a rogue gene in a family breast-cancer sufferer – because she believes Jane would immediately see through such a subterfuge: 'she'd probably have been straight round to Phyllis'. There is little doubt, therefore, that Jane fully appreciates the pivotal position that Phyllis occupies in the dilemma she finds herself in.

The move which Jane makes, to seek out a family member who had hitherto been cut off from the extended family, is one which would very probably take some bravery and determination on her part. But how did Jane communicate with Phyllis when they met? During the meeting, did Jane evince concern only about her own health matters and interests, or did she try to extend the hand of family companionship to Phyllis in expressing concern for her welfare too?

It is notable that Phyllis makes no mention of the meeting with Jane. To the reader this seems surprising as Phyllis has been cut off from her extended family for a decade and a half, and could be expected to have found Jane's approach to her – out of the blue – particularly noteworthy, if only because, in Jane's sudden appearance, Phyllis might perhaps see another example, by a member of Edith's family, of behaviour that was manifestly self-interested. In other words, Phyllis could be expected to have counted Jane's contact as further evidence of her own unacceptable treatment at the hands of her sister's family. But Phyllis fails to refer to the meeting. In the case, the meeting takes place 'behind the scene' and lacks narrative content.

This analysis points to a narrative gap in the composition of the case; what took place between Jane and Phyllis when they met is opaque to the reader.

This gap is unlikely to result from authorial oversight or censorship. A reported remark of Phyllis's betrays *active denial* that a meeting with Jane ever took place: 'I'm not in touch with them' (i.e. other members of the family), a comment attributed to Phyllis by Jane's geneticist. This denial probably means 'whatever contact they wish to have with me I want no contact with them' but it does not rule out further attempts being made, through separate discussions with each, to clarify what actually took place between Jane and Phyllis during their meeting. Jane should be encouraged to examine her motives in seeking out Phyllis, and to reflect on what it could feel like for Phyllis to be approached in this way after a 15-year estrangement. Phyllis should be made aware that members of the medical team, while respecting her point of view and empathising with her isolated situation, deny any legitimacy to blaming her for contracting breast cancer. If Phyllis would allow disclosure, a member of the medical team (possibly the GP), might be able to plead her cause to Jane and other members of the family.

Phyllis should be made aware firmly and sympathetically that precisely by *not* allowing disclosure of her genetic status to interested family members, she will be placing herself in a position in which she could attract blame in the future, once it becomes known (as one day it might) that bilateral mastectomies in relatives who feel forced to seek surgical preventive treatments could have been avoidable if Phyllis had allowed disclosure.

While acknowledging the reasoning behind the well-founded view that 'if counselling does not persuade someone to consent to sharing information with their relatives the individual's decision to withhold information should be paramount' (House of Commons Science and Technology Committee 1995: para. 228) forced interpersonally sophisticated mediation between Jane and Phyllis is one possible solution to the ethical problem posed by this case. Strong encouragement of more dialogue between Phyllis and Jane could enable them to find a way to overcome this impasse.[2]

In whatever way Jane chooses to approach Phyllis again, it is possible that Phyllis will always feel unmoved and unprepared to divulge personal health information to Jane. But it is also possible that Phyllis might mull over the situation, seek reconciliation and change her mind about divulging the relevant information. These possibilities can only be elaborated by deeper, more-layered descriptions of Jane and Phyllis than readers of this account have been offered.

Jane's decision

On returning to the genetics clinic after having 'done loads of reading' and having talked to a familial breast-cancer support group (but having clearly failed to gain Phyllis's confidence), Jane announces she's made a decision. Despite not knowing whether she has, or has not, inherited the familial rogue (BRCA) gene, she has decided she will undergo bilateral mastectomies as prophylaxis against developing breast cancer.[3]

The unseen narrator

The chief narrator of this case history sets out a series of uninterrupted soliloquies on events as they have unfolded. Relationships, communications and many of the events themselves are depicted from the different angles and perspectives of the individuals concerned. Who, then, is the reporting agency of this case history? Excluding the framing of the case (by introduction and author's comment), certain additional clues suggest the presence of Jane's unnamed geneticist. The case presented clearly revolves around Jane as the person in need of advice, testing and possible treatment. Jane's geneticist's clinical responsibility is to Jane, and not Phyllis, and we hear nothing directly from Phyllis's clinical geneticist and little from Phyllis's GP. The coincidence of Jane's geneticist and the case narrator would explain why Phyllis has fewer (and arguably less persuasive) voices representing her interests in the case than does Jane.

We hear from individuals caught up in the scenario in uninterrupted disquisitions from each, with little or no report of argumentation or negotiation taking place *between* them (King and Stanford 1992). The absence of arguments and of actual dialogue that could suggest areas of agreement and disagreement as well as possible resolution, deprives readers of the actual reasoning and personal voices of the dramatis personae of the case, and heightens the sense gained, that each holds fairly fixed ethical positions (perhaps with the exception of the GPs).

As readers, we have to live with the pictures we are presented with. But absence of such elements is part and parcel of a literary deceit that hides the omnipotent role of the narrator in choosing both the means and the manner in which individuals speak out in the case. The narrator is our one and only witness to the events, feelings, reasons and relationships we learn of in the case, and we depend upon the narrator for not omitting, exaggerating or distorting anything important. At the same time, we should realise that no good history or reportage can be written without a measure of imaginative sympathy for those caught up in a story, a sympathy that can convince readers that humans actually acted, thought or felt the way depicted (Ash 2002).

Thus we should appreciate that the analysis engaged in here is a second-order one of interpreting a reconstruction of events, feelings and reasons, presented in the empirical disguise of the words and phrases of participants themselves. This does not annul the ethical problem: Phyllis has information that Jane could benefit from but that Phyllis does not wish to share with Jane, but it helps us to see that the problem confronting us is an elaborate construction embedded in the narrator's rendering of events.

Phyllis's story

In common with Jane, but without explicitly knowing it, Phyllis has come to the same view of the close relationship between her lineage and her likely development of breast cancer. Phyllis's monologue begins in a manner strikingly similar to Jane's self-revelatory opening words. But being older than Jane, Phyllis's intimations of cancer have (sadly) eventuated: 'I knew I was doing pretty well to get to 50 without developing cancer, all the other females in the family had got it much before that, but when I felt the lump in my breast I knew straight away that it was cancer.'

Phyllis then reports that she has had 'the operation'. At around that time she also underwent genetic testing, apparently without actually being asked whether she wished to be genetically tested or not, and without being told that the test results could carry significance for her extended family: 'he just took the blood sample'. Nevertheless, Phyllis recalls discussions with her oncologist, concerning the reasons for such testing, the results of which – she was led to believe – might be of benefit to herself in determining the best treatment of her particular cancer. Phyllis is informed of the test results, which indicate she's positive 'for something'. But in contrast to the rationale offered for genetically testing her, Phyllis is later told that the test results have no bearing on her own treatment, despite the positive result. She is referred to a clinical geneticist – 'the genetic people' – who confirm she does, indeed, carry 'a faulty gene'. However, Phyllis judges her geneticist to be 'wishy-washy', more interested in her family than in herself.

There are many clues here that point to false hopes and expectations, frustrations and false trails on the part of Phyllis and her oncologist. On the surface, Phyllis appears uninterested in detail, purporting not really to know why she was referred ('positive for something') to a clinical geneticist ('the genetic people'). Her response is to tell *her own story* and to tell it in some detail: Phyllis wants her doctors to know that she nursed her mother and sister when they developed breast cancer, has never been thanked for this, and subsequently was cut out of her sister's will and later ignored by her family. Phyllis thereby tells her geneticist (and the reader) what sort of a person she is: a hurt, isolated and stigmatised woman (the picture painted by Phyllis's geneticist whose views in the case are relayed – but how comprehensively? – by

Jane's geneticist). 'So', Phyllis tells us, 'I wasn't happy with them letting others know of my test result.'

Portrayals of Phyllis and Jane

Is there a difference in how Phyllis and Jane have been portrayed in the case history? Phyllis has breast cancer, is alone, grumpy and cut-off from the rest of the family. She appears to be unloving towards her surviving family, possibly unloved, and in her own eyes, blamed; a relatively asocial and marginalised figure. Compare this with the portrayal of Jane, who is depicted as energetic, lively and socially interactive. She is reflective about her responsibilities to her daughters, is supported by family and patient groups, and is in touch with goings-on in the world. Jane is a socially networked person, a loving figure who has a husband to talk to, and a GP and a geneticist who speak up for her.

As mere readers of a text, we can never know how accurately differences in such portrayals within a case transcribe, illuminate or exaggerate real life differences between Phyllis and Jane. But it is important to appreciate that the teller of this tale cannot be an entirely neutral observer of events. As already argued, Jane's clinical geneticist has a duty towards her patient whom she represents in a positive light. By contrast, this narration shows Phyllis to be quite a negative person and to have no-one to turn to for advice and counsel, except perhaps to her GP.

The general practitioners' perspective

The GPs we hear from in the case are in a unique position. They are custodians of Jane's and Phyllis's medical records and of their individual extended clinical histories, and they work together in the same practice partnership. It is Jane's GP whose account we actually hear, and who relates the views of Phyllis's GP: 'My partner [i.e. Phyllis's GP] felt very strongly, and I think I agree with him, that neither we nor anyone else, should break Phyllis's confidentiality.' This sounds like a firm position of principle, one that Phyllis's GP backs up by reference to Phyllis's specific prohibition of disclosure: 'she does not want anyone to know. I think her main reasons are that she would feel blamed by the family and I think that is reasonable.'

Nevertheless, the GP explores the opposite possibility, making reference to the General Medical Council's good practice guidelines, which specify possible exceptions to the rule of medical confidentiality. The guidelines suggest that disclosure can sometimes be the right course of action, even in the face of

specific prohibition, but only where 'a very serious or life-threatening condition' would be likely to eventuate without disclosure and where disclosure
directly concerns a specific, identifiable individual patient for whom the
doctor is medically responsible. Just such a situation pertains in this case
(although Phyllis's GP does not make this point). The genetic information
that the GPs are party to – concerning Phyllis – could help to inform Jane
(and her clinical geneticist) about Phyllis's rogue gene for breast cancer, and
would allow accurate tests on Jane's genetic status to be carried out. If Jane
turned out to be negative for the particular rogue gene, bilateral mastectomy
could be avoided, and Jane would be spared 'a major and mutilating piece of
surgery', the words of her GP concerning this procedure. (In passing, it is
worth noting that divulgence in these circumstances also accords with both
the Nuffield Council's and British Medical Association's views of ethically
correct conduct by GPs) (Nuffield Council on Bioethics 1993: 43, British
Medical Association 1998: 148).[4]

However, in this case history, the GP does *not* appear to consider the full
implications of Jane being positive for the rogue (BRCA) gene. Instead, and
contrary to Jane's clinical geneticist's interpretation of the evidence, the GP
seems to hold that there is insufficient evidence unequivocally to recommend
bilateral mastectomy as an effective preventative manoeuvre against breast
cancer in BRCA-gene-positive individuals. For the GP, since mastectomy
should not (ethically) be offered to Jane, there can be no warrant to breach
Phyllis's medical confidentiality in the face of her specific prohibition.
Instead, the GP supports Jane being offered regular mammography screening, to enable early diagnosis and treatment if and when cancer develops. In
this way, the GP interprets the situation as not falling within one of the
GMC's ethical exceptions that permit breach of confidentiality.

Rather unexpectedly, the GP, towards the end of the testimony, makes a
challenging suggestion about how the situation might best be managed: 'My
partner wondered why they couldn't just test Jane for the gene fault that
they'd found in Phyllis without letting Phyllis know', a course of action
clearly envisaged by the BMA as justifiable in situations such as this one
(British Medical Association 1998: 84).[5] However, in her own mind, the GP
annuls further consideration of this idea by concurring with Jane's geneticist's view, that were this to be undertaken against Phyllis's wishes, Jane
would be placed in a position in which she would infer her aunt's genetic-
test status.

As already indicated, there are strong narrative grounds for believing that
Jane already has an inkling – may implicitly believe – that Phyllis has devel-
oped breast cancer. Without necessarily disclosing anything further about
Phyllis, Jane's GP is in a very good position to gauge Jane's understanding of
Phyllis's situation and to suggest that Jane again talk to Phyllis about her
situation.

The oncologist's story

Unlike that of the GPs, the tone of this clinician's monologue is boisterously defensive, and reads as an apologia seeking to justify genetic tests on Phyllis. The doctor recounts a seminar that had 'suggested' that treatment of hereditary breast and ovarian cancer should be more aggressive than that of sporadic cancer (although Jane's clinical geneticist clearly disagrees with this view, stating there to be no 'good' evidence on this score. Perhaps the seminar was inaccurate or Phyllis's oncologist misread its contents). Nevertheless, the oncologist believed a possible difference in best treatment was the rationale underpinning genetic investigations on Phyllis.

The oncologist's account hints strongly that specific informed consent from Phyllis for the genetic tests was not obtained. He says that Phyllis 'consented to lots of investigative blood tests as part of her diagnosis and treatment' but admits she was not told that these tests, depending upon the results, would carry implications for members of her family. There is a suggestion here that the oncologist appreciates that undertaking genetic tests on Phyllis was morally short-sighted, and that some criticism on this score has been received: 'I realise the genetic-test result has created difficulties'; but her oncologist clings to the conviction that the clinician is ultimately responsible for the patient, and patient autonomy would be compromised by offering relatives a say in whether or not genetic tests are undertaken. Whatever the quality of the evidence relied on, the oncologist subsequently perceives that there could be a family interest in this information, although no mention of Jane or her situation is made in this doctor's account.

What does the oncologist's account contribute to the case history? It offers no view on the nub of the dilemma facing Jane's geneticist and her GP, and it is possible that Phyllis's oncologist does not even know of Jane's existence. However, the oncologist's account provides the narrative link that explains why and how (without informed consent) Phyllis came to be genetically tested in the first place. It also reveals how her test results came to be made available to Jane's clinical geneticist. The oncologist thereby offers a convincing account of how the ethical issue about whether to divulge Phyllis's health information to Jane actually came to arise.

The geneticist's story

As with the GP account in this case history, the geneticist we hear from has clinical responsibility for Jane and not for Phyllis. Jane's doctor's account provides much of the factual genetic detail Jane was given when she first attended the genetics service, and on which she based her decision to seek out Phyllis and later to request mastectomy. Jane's geneticist relays the views of Phyllis's geneticist, that Phyllis 'is a sad and isolated lady who shouldn't be bullied into doing something she thinks will bring her harm'. Jane's geneticist discusses the possibility of 'fudging' the issue with Jane, going back on the original explanation she first gave Jane and telling her that a genetic test can now be performed without the use of genetic information from an affected family member. But she decides against this course of action – designed to avoid explicit contravention of Phyllis's prohibition of disclosure of her genetic status – on the grounds that it would, in fact, amount to just that, as Jane (in her view) would be bound to guess from where the required information had come.

Jane's geneticist's view is that Phyllis's test result 'really belongs to her whole family' and that for this reason genetic testing should generally only be undertaken with agreement to disclosure to interested family members agreed as a precondition. However, in this particular case (and generally at the present time), this was not the agreed basis of the test undertaken on Phyllis, so Jane's geneticist does not seek to justify disclosure to Jane on this basis. Instead, Jane's geneticist concludes that her professional responsibility to protect Jane from suffering the harm that bilateral mastectomy would represent – which offers Jane (in the view of her geneticist) little or no benefit if Jane is not a rogue gene carrier – trumps her responsibility, as a doctor and co-professional of Phyllis's geneticist, to respect Phyllis's medical confidentiality. Jane's geneticist decides, therefore, that she would tell Jane about Phyllis's test result and ensure that Phyllis be advised of this 'in as sensitive a way as possible'.

Closure

This case shows how clinical medicine can be both a response to narrative episodes in people's lives and a constitutive part of further episodes in the lives of family members. (Morgan 2001: 5) Traditional analysis in medical ethics, it has been argued, 'rushed to generalise about "the patient", "the subject", "the doctor" and "the researcher"' and strained for principles and universals, while paying insufficient attention to the specificity of individuals, groups and their contexts (Wolf 1986). Ethical analyses also paid too little attention to the storied nature of moral quandaries, and the manner and means by which events, emotions and actions are emplotted in case histories (Hurwitz 2000, Greenhalgh and Hurwitz 1998). As the novelist Flannery O'Connor once wrote: 'a story is a way to say something that can't be said any other way. You tell a story because a statement would be inadequate' (O'Connor 1972).

This genetics case is just such a story. It ends with Jane's geneticist concluding that she *would* disclose Phyllis's medical details to Jane, against Phyllis's wishes, but not that she *has already done so*. Use of the subjunctive tense, here, allows the manner and reasoning behind closure of this tale to be clearly formulated and sketched out, while final closure is left for the reader to accomplish.

Whatever Phyllis is like in real life, a close reading of the case indicates that the portrayal does not rhetorically balance Phyllis's interests with those of Jane's. Jane's geneticist's conclusion – that the wrong (and possible harm) that Phyllis would suffer if her confidentiality is breached is outweighed by the prevention of harm that could be achieved by preventing Jane from undergoing unnecessary mastectomy – means that Jane's interests should win out over those of Phyllis. But why should Jane's geneticist so completely reject subterfuge (the 'fudging' solution)? Whether or not Jane would be able to guess the provenance of genetic information used to test her for BRCA status – and a narrative reading suggests that she would guess it correctly – its origin needs no further discussion, confirmation or denial on the part of Jane's geneticist or GP. Such a fudge would require professional silence to be maintained, and arguably would cause least harm to each party.[5] However, a fudge of this sort would require Jane's geneticist, in going back on her word, to deal directly and perhaps uncomfortably with Jane. Jane's geneticist opts, instead, for a solution that requires Phyllis be told of the disclosure but by other (unspecified) doctors. In the real world this solution would require the cooperation of Phyllis's GP and geneticist, neither of whom appear to support this solution. Indeed, Phyllis's and Jane's GPs quite explicitly oppose such a solution.

How does Jane's geneticist propose dealing with the likely opposition of the GPs to her proposed strategy? What would Jane's geneticist do if Phyllis's geneticist disagreed too, and refused to play a part in her plan? These considerations indicate that the solution proposed by Jane's geneticist, and the plan suggested for its implementation, may not work in the way envisaged.

Conclusion

Stories are a foundational means of depicting people, their vicissitudes and experiences. Narrative analysis in healthcare usually arises from the need to make sense of transcribed interviews and assumes narratives, however fragmentary, constitute the social reality of interviewees. Such analysis is formally text based, and proceeds on extended segments of transcribed talk in a way not possible in the case of Jane and Phyllis, because their thoughts and feelings are not made available to us in their own words. In this situation, a formal narrative analysis is therefore not possible. However, analysis of the narrative in this case is possible, and highlights the following features of Jane and Phyllis's dilemma worthy of attention and action in the real word of clinical practice:

- the importance of recognising who is narrating an ethics case, the narrative devices the teller employs, and the determinative influences narrators can exert on how readers respond to a moral dilemma;
- the contrast manifest in this case, between the positive depiction of Jane as a much more fully rounded figure than Phyllis, who is portrayed as a partial, isolated and marginalised figure;
- the consonance in the case, between Jane's positive presence and the first person appearances of her medical advocates in the case – her own GP and clinical geneticist – and the negative portrayal of Phyllis who has to make do with the views of her GP and geneticist being reported secondhand by Jane's doctors;
- the strong likelihood that Jane already believes, or at the very least has strong suspicions, that Phyllis has developed breast cancer (albeit Jane cannot know, without being told, whether such a cancer has a genetic or sporadic basis);
- that a narrative gap in the case is identified – concerning what happened when Jane met Phyllis – and stands in need of clarification. Jane's GP (or geneticist) should suggest to Jane that she examine her motives for seeking out Phyllis after a 15-year estrangement, and that Jane reflect on what it could feel like for Phyllis to be approached by her in this way;
- that Phyllis should be approached by her GP or geneticist to discuss the consequences for Phyllis's surviving family (Jane, her daughters and future unborn individuals), of Phyllis's refusal to disclose her genetic status to them. The discussion should concentrate on reassuring Phyllis that she cannot be blamed for developing breast cancer, and that were she to inform Jane of her genetic status, the clinicians would help to ensure that Phyllis's breast cancer is seen in the light of the family lineage of which it is an expression, for which Phyllis cannot meaningfully be blamed. Such discussion could help Phyllis to see that the possible consequences of bilateral mastectomies on the physical, psychological and sexual well-being of relatives, who are forced to seek surgery in an attempt to prevent breast cancer, could more legitimately result in Phyllis's attracting the very blame she wishes to avoid.

The philosopher Jonathan Glover has argued that ethics as a discipline cannot be practised and advanced without a sophisticated appreciation of people (Glover 1999: 6). Forced mediation between Jane and Phyllis is the narrative solution to the ethical problem posed by this case, but the only chance it stands of success will depend on how sensitively such mediation attends to the needs and personalities of Jane and Phyllis themselves. But how forced should forced mediation be? Aristotle theorised tragedy as a well-constructed view of events and actions unified by a plot in which all the parts and characters work inexorably, whether consciously or not, toward an unavoidable end. If Jane cannot be made to understand Phyllis, and Phyllis remains obdurate despite attempts to help her to see the consequences for her extended family, the case will take on some of the hallmarks of a tragedy. Either Phyllis is to be wronged through infringement of her privacy and medical confidentiality, or Jane is to be avoidably harmed by allowing her to seek potentially unnecessary surgery. If forced mediation fails, then the issue surely should be fudged by offering Jane the genetic test she needs without divulging the source of the genetic information. This subterfuge would avoid a formal breach of Phyllis's confidentiality, and would allow surgery to be avoided if Jane proves BRCA-gene negative.

ACKNOWLEDGEMENT

Many thanks to Ruth Richardson and Hazel McHaffie for helpful discussion about this case.

NOTES

1 If Jane's mother, Edith, had had a 'rogue' gene (had been heterozygous for a BRCA gene, a worst-case scenario) she understands there would be a 50% chance that she, Jane, would have inherited such a gene, making it very likely that she will develop breast cancer. In the absence of precise knowledge of the nature of the rogue gene's many possible (allelic) forms – which can be detected in Jane only if the results of genetic tests on a known breast cancer sufferer in Jane's family are utilised – the screening tests currently available are neither sufficiently sensitive nor specific to delineate her risk of carrying the relevant gene. But in the context of detailed genetic information from a family sufferer of breast cancer, a screening test on Jane would be much more effective in estimating her risk of developing the disease, because it would offer a result with a high degree of certainty concerning her likelihood of having inherited the rogue (BRCA) gene for cancer. This set of facts is presented in Jane's geneticist's account.

2 There are indications from Jane's clinical geneticist's account that a further meeting between Jane and Phyllis has already been suggested: 'my colleague [that is, Phyllis's geneticist, whose account we only hear in this way] has tried hard to suggest to Phyllis that it would be in the interest of her family to disclose ... but she just doesn't see it as in her best interest ... She shouldn't be bullied into doing something she thinks will bring her harm.'

3 There is little indication from the case as to whether this decision by Jane is likely to be considered a real treatment option by Jane's doctors, and a future surgeon asked to consider Jane's request sits strictly outside the framework of this analysis. But questions such as:

- can a surgeon be found who would be prepared to remove the apparently healthy breasts of a 36-year-old woman as a prophylactic procedure against a (so-far) undefined risk of developing cancer?

- what would be the reduction in absolute risk of Jane developing breast cancer if she underwent mastectomies, on the one hand if she has the rogue gene in question, and on the other hand if she were free of this rogue gene?
- if Jane is referred for bilateral mastectomy, should the referring GP or geneticist divulge that Jane, in fact, has an aunt, who unbeknown to Jane, carries the relevant BRCA gene?
- could a surgeon be made liable for agreeing to perform an operation that non-negligently leads to harm, say, were Jane to suffer complications such as recurrent breakdown of wounds and chest-wall abscesses, which ruin her quality of life and lead to the break-up of her marriage, if it could later be proven that Jane was in fact free of the BRCA gene (Phyllis might change her mind and enable Jane to be diagnostically tested)?

raise issues to be weighed in deciding whether this sort of preventative treatment in Jane's circumstances can be considered ethical. The seriousness with which Jane's clinical geneticist views her request is indicated by her reference to a lack of professional consensus on the wisdom of such surgery in Jane's case, to the 'accumulating evidence that the lifetime risk of cancer following such an operation is significantly reduced' and to the lack of 'any data that suggest the mortality from breast cancer is reduced if these women have such an operation'.

4 Nuffield Council on Bioethics (1993). *Genetics Screening: Ethical Issues*. London: Nuffield Council, 43. 'In exceptional circumstances, health professionals might be justified in disclosing genetic information to other family members, despite an individual's desire for confidentiality.' British Medical Association (1998). *Human Genetics*. London: BMA, 148. 'There may be rare cases in which, despite being informed of the relevance of the information to other family members, the patient refuses to raise the issue with other relatives at risk or to consent to anyone else approaching them . . . it may be decided that the level of risk of harm to the patient's parent, children, or siblings would be sufficiently high to justify disclosure to those people . . . These decisions will usually be made by the Regional Genetics Centre, preferably in consultation with the patient's GP. Before any information is disclosed, the patient should be informed of the intention to divulge the information and to whom and the reasons why such action is considered justified . . . If the patient and the person or people to be contacted have the same GP, the BMA believes that their GP would be the most appropriate person to make the disclosure . . . '

5 British Medical Association (1998: 84). 'In some exceptional cases disclosure of information, without consent, will be justified. Wherever possible information should be passed to relatives in a way that does not identify the patient. This might be done by simply informing the individual that information has been obtained from "a relative" without naming the person or relationship.'

REFERENCES

Ash, T. G. (2002). Truth is another country. *The Guardian*, Review, 16 November, 4–6. http://books.guardian.co.uk/

Booth, W. (2002). Ethics of medicine, as revealed in literature. In R. Charon and M. Montello, eds. *Stories Matter*. New York and London: Routledge.

British Medical Association. (1998). *Human Genetics*. London: BMA.

Chambers, T. S. (1994). The bioethicist as author: the medical ethics case as rhetorical device. *Lit Med*, **13**, 60–78.

 (1999). *The Fiction of Bioethics: Cases as Literary Texts*. New York: Routledge.

 (2002). From the ethicist's point of view: the literary nature of ethical enquiry. *Hastings Center Report* Jan.–Feb. 1996. Reproduced in K. W. M. (Bill) Fulford, D. L. Dickenson and T. H. Murray, *Healthcare Ethics and Human Values*. Cambridge: CUP, 70–5.

Cobley, P. (2001). *Narrative*. London: Routledge.

Forster, E. M. (1971). *Aspects of the Novel*. Harmondsworth, Middx: Penguin Books.

Glover, J. (1999). *Humanity: A Moral History of the Twentieth Century*. London: Jonathan Cape.

Greenhalgh, T. and Hurwitz, B., eds., (1998). *Narrative-Based Medicine*. London: BMJ Books.

Guroian, V. (1998). *Tending the Heart of Virtue*. Oxford: OUP.

House of Commons Science and Technology Committee. (1995). *Human Genetics: The Science and Its Consequences*. London: HMSO.

Hurwitz, B. (2000). Narrative and the practice of medicine. *Lancet*, **356**, 2086–9.

 (2002). Informed consent and access to personal medical records for the purposes of health services research. In L. Doyal and J. Tobias, eds., *Informed Consent in Medical Research*. London: BMJ Books, 230–9.

King, N. M. P. and Stanford, A. F. (1992). Patient stories, doctor stories, and true stories: a cautionary reading. *Lit Med*, **11**, 185–99.

Levine, P. (1998). *Living Without Philosophy: On Narrative, Rhetoric, and Morality*. Albany: State University of New York Press.

MacIntyre, A. (1981). *After Virtue: A Study in Moral Theory*. London: Duckworth.

Morgan, D. (2001). *Issues in Medical Law and Ethics*. London: Cavendish.

Nuffield Council on Bioethics. (1993). *Genetics Screening: Ethical Issues*. London: Nuffield Council.

O'Connor, F. (1972). *Mystery and manners: Occasional Prose*. Selected and edited by S. Fitzgerald and R. Fitzgerald. London: Faber & Faber.

Pellegrino, E. D. (1997). Bioethics as an interdisciplinary enterprise: where does ethics fit in the mosaic of disciplines? In R. A. Carson and C. R. Burns, eds., *Philosophy of Medicine and Bioethics*. Dordrecht: Kluwer, 1–23.

Smith, H. B. (1981). Narrative versions, narrative theories. In W. J. T. Mitchell, ed., *On Narrative*. Chicago: University of Chicago Press, 209–32.

Uspensky, B. (1973). *A Poetics of Composition*. Berkeley: University of California Press.

Walzer, M. (1987). *Interpretation and Social Criticism*. Cambridge, Mass.: Harvard University Press.

Widdowshoven, G. A. M. and Smits, M. -J. (1996). Ethics and narratives. In R. Josselson, ed., *Ethics and Process in the Narrative Study of Lives*, vol. 4. Newburypark: Sage, 275–87.

Widdershoven, G. and Sohl, C. (1999). Interpretation, communication and action. Four stories about supported employment. In T. A. Abma, ed., *Telling Tales; On Evaluation and Narrative*. *Advances in Program Evaluation*, Vol. 6. Greenwich, Conn.: JAI Press 109–130.

Wolf, S. M. (1986). *Feminism and Bioethics*. New York: OUP.

4

A virtue-ethics approach

Alastair Campbell

Introducing virtue ethics

Perhaps the simplest way of understanding the basic approach of virtue ethics to moral problems is to adopt the contrast suggested by Crisp (1996). Modern moral philosophy, heavily influenced by the philosophy of Immanuel Kant and by the rival theories of the Utilitarians, has tended to focus on the question 'How should I *act*?' but the resurgence of virtue ethics is a return to a more ancient question 'How should I *live*?'. This marks a shift from an ethics of obligation (*deontic* ethics) based on universal principles or rules to an ethics of character (*areteic* ethics) based on an account of virtue. In virtue ethics the main focus is therefore not individual actions but the *character* of the moral agent.

Statman (1997) offers a full analysis of the range of possibilities in this renewed emphasis on character as the foundation of morality. *Moderate* approaches to virtue ethics, he suggests, regard it as complementary to action-based approaches. On this approach, virtue cannot be subsumed under the notion of following moral rules – it has its distinctive place in a full understanding of morality. This full understanding does equally require an account of rule-based universal obligations, but by adding judgements of character to judgements of right action we get a richer account than either offers separately. *Radical* approaches to virtue ethics, by contrast, do not accept this complementarity: in such approaches, judgements of character are always seen as prior to judgements of action. In *reductionist radical* virtue ethics the force of statements of rightness or obligatoriness is derived from their source in the actions of a virtuous character; in *replacement radical* virtue ethics deontic statements are rejected altogether – they may even be seen to have a pernicious effect on morality. In this most radical approach all that counts is the presence or absence of virtue. (Alasdair MacIntyre's total rejection of the post-Enlightenment project in *After Virtue* could be seen as a powerful example of this replacement approach.)

Case Analysis in Clinical Ethics, ed. Richard Ashcroft, Anneke Lucassen, Michael Parker, Marian Verkerk, Guy Widdershoven. Published by Cambridge University Press.
© Cambridge University Press 2005.

In bioethics, virtue ethics is yet to have a major influence, and as I shall note below it has tended to be restricted to attempts to describe the characteristics of the virtuous professional. The dominant principlist approach to bioethics (see, for example, Gillon in this book) has reversed the reductionist approach described above: for the principlist, the virtues are relevant to morality but only if they are derivative from universal moral principles. For example, Gillon (1994: 330) writes:

> Descriptions, such as wise, brave, tolerant, persevering, dependable, sincere, loyal, humorous, humble, open, warm, are all character descriptions. But whether or not they are to be described as virtuous will surely depend on the extent to which they tend to produce morally desirable attitudes and behaviour ... whether or not they tend to respect autonomy, be beneficial, avoid harming, and be just.

In a similar vein Beauchamp and Childress (1994), while including virtue ethics in this later edition of their influential book, reject the idea that virtue can be the prior measure of morality: 'It is unacceptable to claim that if persons display a virtuous character, their acts are therefore morally acceptable' (p. 68). However, in what they call a 'constructive evaluation of character ethics' (p. 69) they do concede that ethical theory may be more complete if the virtues are included. Here, in the terminology of Statman, they seem to be agreeing with the moderate approach to virtue ethics, which sees separate and complementary roles for deontic and areteic theories.

In this chapter I too am adopting a moderate approach to the question of the relationship between principlism and other theories. I certainly do not wish to replace principles totally with assessments of character, but neither do I accept the idea that principles are in some way logically prior to virtue, as Gillon seems to imply. Questions of moral attitudes, of settled ways of relating to moral concerns or, in the phrase of Robert Bellah (1985), 'habits of the heart' are, in my view, critical issues for bioethics, and they are easily overlooked if we always start with an analysis of moral problems in terms of principles. We need a separate assessment of what is going on in moral dilemmas like the one described in the case study in Chapter 1, which starts and finishes with an account of virtue. However, before attempting to relate virtue ethics to the case study, it is important to consider some common criticisms of the approach and the response that virtue ethics could make to these. Four problems are often identified both by external critics and by proponents of virtue ethics itself:

1. that the assessment of virtue is entirely culture-specific and so of no use in a general account of morality;
2. that virtues are supererogatory and so a use of them will lead to elitism and stigmatisation;
3. that the notion of virtue is too broad and non-specific to allow for practical application;

4. that an emphasis on the moral character of individuals ignores social and
   communal dimensions.

In what follows I shall address each of these in turn.

Cultural relativity

This is the most common criticism of virtue ethics. As Aristotle is often
regarded as the father of virtue ethics (some would say wrongly; see Simpson
1997), the limitations of his account are seen as fatal. Aristotle saw virtue
epitomised in the Athenian gentle*man*. The traits he described seem to
epitomise the prejudices of upper-class males in a society that accepted
slavery and the alleged inferiority of women. How then can this form the
basis of a universal ethic? In an important paper, Nussbaum (1988) has
effectively confronted this criticism. She argues that we can identify a set of
non-relative virtues, which relate to universal aspects of human experience,
such as birth, love, illness and death. These virtues cohere in a general
understanding of human flourishing, but just how they will be expressed in
practice will vary according to cultural and historical circumstances – an
obvious example will be differing attitudes to illness and death. Thus there
are universal virtues, but they are 'thin', basic forms of human attitudes to
non-optional events. They acquire 'thickness' according to their social and
cultural context and so we may reasonably expect variation from society to
society and epoch to epoch. This variation, however, does not prevent us
from asking whether the particular cultural form aids or inhibits human
flourishing. Hence we may criticise alleged virtues if, for example, they
encourage disregard of particular social groups.

Critics may not be fully persuaded by this response. They may ask, whence
comes this concept of 'human flourishing'? Is it transhistorical, culturally
non-specific? To this the virtue ethicist must reply that there are certain
intrinsic human goods that cannot be ultimately demonstrated – either we
recognise them or we do not. In this respect, the defence goes on, *all* ethical
theory depends on the acceptance without further proof of certain fundamental perceptions. The proponent of the Four Principles theory, for example, cannot prove that these are fundamental or universally recognised.
Equally we may claim that the basic features of the virtuous character,
which result in a rounded human life, are universally perceived, but cannot
be proved. (This is sometimes called the 'partners in crime' defence!)

Elitism and stigma

The second criticism may be seen as a misunderstanding of the approach. To
describe virtues as supererogatory is to attempt to force virtue ethics into a
deontic straitjacket. The theory is not an account of obligation but of the

growth and consistency of particular traits of character. It is a contradiction in terms to say that a person is obliged to be virtuous, for, if he or she feels obliged, he or she is not virtuous, merely pretending to be! Conversely, a person who lacks, say, generosity or courage, may simply be incapable of these virtues for whatever reasons that have led to the formation of their character to date. Of course this raises some tricky problems for moral theory, captured in the phrase 'moral luck' (see Parfit 1984), but these are hardly a problem only for virtue ethics. We simply do not fully understand why it is easier for some persons than others to lead the moral life. Those who fail, whether by deontic or areteic criteria, may well be blamed, just as morally good actions and character are often praised. But such praise or blame may be at best only partly fair. From the virtue-ethics perspective, the point of describing virtue is not to single out some elite class or to stigmatise the unworthy. On the contrary, virtue ethics aims to describe everyday features of the moral life, easily recognisable in everyone, not some attributes of *Übermenschen*. By offering such descriptions virtue ethics seeks to enable character formation, for role models are an important source of education in virtue.

On the other hand, it has to be said that the virtue-ethics approach can become elitist. This has been a problem in bioethics, since much of the early literature focused on the virtuous physician (see May 1983, 1991; Pellegrino and Thomasma 1998). The result has been a tendency to idealise the professional and to ignore the fact that the patient is the principal actor in the healthcare encounter (see Campbell 1998). In a recently completed research project, I and my other European colleagues have sought to redress this balance with a stress on the virtues of patients (Campbell and Swift 2002).

Applicability

Does virtue ethics help with practical situations like the one we are discussing in this book? The question may be better answered later when I relate the approach to the case, but in general terms one may say that whether a theory is applicable is itself a value judgement. Virtue ethics (even in its most radical form) does not seek to produce specific action guides of the kind attempted by principle-based theories. Virtue ethics is concerned more with the ongoing narrative than with the critical moment of decision ('How shall I live?', not 'How shall I act?'). It discusses enduring traits of character rather than specific choices. For example, in the research referred to in the last section we found that people with chronic illness needed a set of character traits, including realism and a sense of humour, in order to maintain a sense of self-worth through an irremediable and often demoralising experience of pain and disability. How they made decisions at particular moments was of concern to them, certainly, but the bigger challenge was to persevere through years of struggle to remain a person valued by others and by themselves.

Because virtue ethics is orientated towards attitudes rather than actions it could be more applicable to a majority of patients than an action-oriented theory. The 'high-tech' medical emergency (so beloved of the media) is only a small part of bioethics.

Self and community

Finally I need to consider whether virtue ethics tends towards individualism. There is no doubt that it is a highly personalised approach, indeed that is one of its central features. In contrast with the notion of a set of formal universal principles (like those of Beauchamp and Childress), virtue ethics stresses features of the individual moral life. Moreover, moral character is not static or timeless. Over time my character is formed by numerous incidents and influences and it may well change radically in response to major traumatic events in my later life. (See May 1991 for a vivid account of this in relation to the Dax case.) Also, unlike principlism, virtue ethics does not deal exclusively with relationships with others. It is concerned with self-regarding as well as with other-regarding virtues. It encourages questions of the form, what sort of person do I want to be? What sort of person have I become? In this respect, it may be seen to be similar to some forms of religious quest. Some questions in medical ethics seem particularly appropriate to these aspects of virtue ethics; for example, the choices of patients to refuse some potentially life-prolonging treatments or the concept of 'dying well'.

Is it true, then, that virtue ethics ignores the communal and social dimensions of ethics? Some writers in the field would strenuously deny this. For example, MacIntyre's account of the intrinsic good of practices and of the moral quest is essentially communal. (This is discussed more fully in the next section.) Clearly there is an intimate relationship between virtue and culture as I observed earlier, but while culture may form the 'thickness' of virtue, it is less obvious that virtue can change the very thing that forms it. In this respect deontic theories, with their claims to overarching moral principles, seem a more likely source of criticism. Yet the intriguing question remains of whether virtuous people are not by the very dynamics of their characters, by the nature of the questions they ask themselves and others, agents for change. In this sense virtue ethics might be seen to be subtly sociopolitical.

The case study

When I start to consider the specific case study, I am faced with an immediate problem. Unlike principlism, with its famous 'Georgetown Mantra' of the Four Principles, there is no standard terminology in modern virtue ethics. There are, of course, plenty of lists of virtues in the tradition, notably the 'cardinal virtues' of temperance, courage, prudence and justice, originating from Plato, to which Aquinas added the 'theological virtues' of faith, hope and love, based on the teaching of 1 Corinthians 13. Christian tradition, in the service of penitential practice and moral education, offered a corresponding list of vices, most famously the seven 'deadly sins' of pride, covetousness, lust, gluttony, envy, anger and sloth. Aristotle provided a different set of categories. Relating virtue to the fulfilment of one's proper task or purpose, he saw human fulfilment or happiness (*eudaimonia*) as a blend of intellectual virtues and moral virtues (the rational control of desire). The difference between virtue and vice was determined by the 'golden mean', a balance between excess and deficit in the exercise of desire.

Modern writing in virtue ethics tends to avoid list-making, for the obvious reason, referred to earlier, that such lists can be very culturally determined. (For example, seeing anger as a deadly sin can overlook some very useful ways in which this emotion leads to honest communication and social change; see Campbell 1984.) Now it is more common to describe a general orientation towards the evaluation of learned habits and attitudes that aid the moral life. Examples of these are the notion of a balance of self-regarding and other-regarding virtues, the account by MacIntyre of a narrative quest in which small communities find together the value of 'practices', and the continuing use of the Aristotelian notion of *eudaimonia* to assess the presence or absence of virtue. In the analysis that follows I shall use these more general accounts rather than the traditional listing of virtues.

I begin with Jane's story. At first glance, it might seem like a decisional dilemma. How should she act? Should she have the radical mastectomy or not? (Incidentally, it is not obvious how principlism would answer such a dilemma, except to aver that her autonomy must be respected.) But while it is true that Jane must make this hard choice sooner or later, the moral issues are much richer and more complex. Jane has to learn to live with the knowledge, which she describes as a 'gnawing anxiety', that she is part of a family in which breast cancer is a constant threat. She lives with the memory of her own mother's death, when she herself was only 21, and with fears for her own daughters, that either they may suffer a similar bereavement or themselves be victims of the disease. Clearly, too, Jane's relationship with her husband is an open and mutually supportive one, and so her attitude toward the potential disease and ways of dealing with it is partly formed in ongoing discussion with him. Add to all this, the fact that Jane is intelligent and well informed and so is well able to understand the scientific uncertainty in possible genetic predictions and we begin to see the magnitude of the challenge that she faces.

At this point we can note that virtue ethics has much in common with narrative ethics (see, for example, Hurwitz in this book). It is opposed to a narrowing of perspective to a single decisional moment, with some general moral principle to be appealed to or some conflict of principles to be resolved. Rather, virtue ethics looks to Jane's strengths of character, formed over many years of living with this knowledge. How shall she live with such tragic uncertainty and such hard choices? How can she make her life into something less anxiety-prone and more fulfilling than her current lying awake and fretting in the early hours? In response to such questions, virtue ethics might offer the concept of a balance of self- and other-regarding virtues. It is obvious that for Jane her immediate family is of the highest importance and her more distant family a source of continuing pain. She wants the best for her husband and children, she grieves for her mother and their lack of communication and she regrets the tense relationship with her aunt. Some of this she can resolve, on the basis of the information she currently has, some she must learn to live with, as a reality she cannot change. To have her own breasts surgically removed is a major price to pay for the strengthening of her capacity to be a loving mother and wife, but she seems to be moving that way, and to do this is to seek that balance of concern for herself (in resolving anxiety) and her full participation in her immediate family. To help her in this she has another community of shared experience and value to turn to, the mastectomy support group. Should she have the operation, the challenges will not, of course, end. Although she will probably avoid cancer herself, she will not be sure about her daughters' future. From a virtue-ethics perspective, what will stand her in good stead here will be the habits of realism and honesty she has learned in her life, in contrast with her mother's denial of communication. When her children are older, honest and considerate communication will be the next way in which the virtues she has learned the hard way will be exercised.

Would all this change for Jane if the doctors decided to breach confidentiality and test her for the rogue gene associated with her aunt's cancer? Here the science is complicated, but, as I understand it, considerable uncertainty would remain, unless it were definitely shown that Jane had the same rogue gene. The absence of this gene would not itself be a guarantee that she is 'safe', partly because the testing techniques could yield a false negative and partly because other mutations could be responsible. If this is so, then Jane would still be left with anxiety and would still be wondering about mastectomy. Moreover, she would have the (presumably unwelcome) knowledge that her aunt had had the cancer but had kept the news from her. This alternative scenario would certainly call on the same reserves of character in Jane as the current one.

Turning to Phyllis, the aunt, one can see how a simplistic version of virtue ethics might easily stigmatise her. Is she the villain of the piece? How can her bitterness and fear of blame lead her to act in such a selfish way, refusing to consider the potential benefit she might confer on her niece and grandnieces? However, a virtue-ethics approach based on *eudaimonia* would not engage in blame of this kind – ironically it is blame that she already fears! Instead it seeks to understand the nature of Phyllis's character and to see how it seems to have developed and where it is leading her. Like Jane she has experienced both loss and the fear of cancer, but both to a greater degree. She had learned to expect cancer, which she in fact got, but now must be aware that recurrence cannot be ruled out. She lived through the deaths of both her mother and sister, nursing them when they were dying. Jane regrets the lack of honesty from her mother, but for Phyllis it was much worse: she feels used and abused. The anger at the way she was treated is still very much present with her and she sees herself vulnerable to further attack by a family that regards her (she believes) as the source of all its trouble. So her way of relating to people is to be self-contained, brusque and realistic about her own condition, while seeing it as her business and nobody else's.

It is often a temptation to want to change people like Phyllis, to wish that they had not reacted to earlier traumas by closing themselves down so much, trying to avoid further hurt by exposing as little of themselves as possible to human contact. But virtue ethics is not about sudden changes of character: no Damascus road conversions! It is about the gradual formation of habits of the heart, which lead to a greater or lesser extent to our fulfilment as individuals living in community. Perhaps we may judge that Phyllis, as a result of her unhappy experiences, is unfulfilled, grumpy, paranoid even. But such judgements from outside the individual's own experiences are always dubious. She may see herself as perfectly content and have no wish to change. Virtue ethics cannot by its nature impose obligations on her to change, and certainly can provide no basis for insisting that she ought to allow her information to be shared with her niece. In this regard, the temptations of the doctors to bully her into doing it or to do it behind her back are utterly misplaced. Such moves would merely confirm her view that people are against her.

The only route for an areteic ethic is one of encouragement and of role modelling, which may allow the person to begin to change their acquired ways of relating to others. What might happen, for example, if Jane were to visit her aunt once more, but this time to share her dilemma about the mastectomy and her worries about her daughters' futures? What if she were to ask her aunt's advice, as someone who must surely herself feared the onset of cancer? The result could be a similar rebuff, but at least Phyllis has been given the opportunity to move from self-absorption to seeing the need of others for her help. It might open a new path in the development of her character.

Finally we must consider the roles played by the health professionals in this case. I have deliberately left them till last because, as I observed earlier, too much ink has been spilled describing the virtues of health professionals while ignoring those of patients. The principal story is that of Jane, her daughters and her aunt. The various doctors and scientists appear at critical moments but they are not the lead characters, much as they might think so at times. Long after they have forgotten about their worries about confidentiality and about policy in genetic testing raised by this case, the family will still be living with an inheritance of a virulent and often fatal disease. Given these caveats, we still have to ask about the virtue-ethics perspective on the various professional actions and attitudes. For this task the most useful terminology may be that of MacIntyre, in his description of 'practices'. Here is how he defines a practice (in language that is typically convoluted!):

> By a 'practice' I am going to mean any coherent and complex form of socially established cooperative human activity through which goods internal to that form of activity are realized in the course of trying to achieve those standards of excellence which are appropriate to, and partially derivative of, that form of activity, with the result that human powers to achieve excellence, and human conceptions of the ends and goods involved, are systematically extended. (MacIntyre 1985: 187)

MacIntyre goes on to observe that the goods inherent to any practice can only be realized 'by subordinating ourselves within the practice in our relationship to other practitioners' (p. 191). In other words practices must be cooperative and each member of the group must learn with others and without excessive individualism. A virtue can now be defined as 'an acquired human quality, the possession and exercise of which tends to enable us to achieve those goods which are internal to practices . . . ' (MacIntyre 1985: 191).

There are at least two practices in a MacIntyrean sense in our scenario, that of medicine and that of science. There might be an argument for saying that they are part of the same practice but I think this would ignore certain key issues, which emerge if we separate them. The goods internal to medicine are clearly such things as the diagnosis and therapy of disease and the forming of relationships with patients that aid in their recovery or enable them to cope with the suffering of irremediable conditions. Goods internal to science, on the other hand, consist of the sustained and honest pursuit of knowledge, a spirit of enquiry, which seeks innovative solutions, toleration of uncertainty and openness to rebuttal of accepted views.

The practice of medicine is illustrated in two different groups in this scenario: the general practitioners and the specialist oncologist. For the former the moral challenge comes from the need to maintain, with both Jane and Phyllis, an ongoing therapeutic relationship and at the same time provide them with the best available advice about treatment options. The stumbling block is the requirement of confidentiality, which prevents giving Jane access to the full range of information that both practitioners (accidentally) now possess. They seek to resolve this problem by reference to professional rules, promulgated by the General Medical Council, but unhappy with the conclusion this brings (no immediate threat to life requiring a breach), they think of a way round the rule! But from a virtue-ethics perspective such a device is not possible. One of the goods internal to medicine is the relationship of trust between practitioner and patient, which enables therapy and continuing care to be effective. The corresponding professional virtue is fidelity. Both women face a lifetime of uncertainty about the onset or recurrence of cancer in themselves or their family. They need practitioners who are utterly trustworthy and, although Jane might be relieved to get some further way of assessing her need of a mastectomy, the mode of its discovery (which could not realistically be concealed from her) will lead her to question how secure her own personal information might be in that general practice. It is worth noting that this is not just a consequentialist argument. Virtues are related to intrinsic goods, not instrumental goods. So, even if one could be sure that the breach of confidence would never be discovered, the failure of professional fidelity would still be a major deficit from a virtue-ethics perspective.

Phyllis also met a different medical practitioner, a 'young and energetic' oncologist. His action caused some raised eyebrows among the geneticists, since he appears to have taken blood for testing without adequate consent and sent it off to the genetics service without exploring the implications with Phyllis first. As a result Phyllis felt she had been rushed into something and she wanted no part in it beyond any information affecting her directly. Since specialists, such as the oncologist, have more episodic contacts with patients, focused on a specific condition in which they are experts, they may more easily miss out on the relationship aspect of the internal goods of medicine. Moreover, they may not be so good at 'subordinating themselves' to relationships with other practitioners in the practice. Widdershoven and Weijts (2002) offer us a terminology for understanding what may have been going on here. In an essay on diagnostic styles in clinical relationships they describe three contrasting styles – rationalist, relativist and dialogical – and compare them with the detective styles of Poirot, William of Baskerville and Maigret. The Poirot style is deductive and it assumes a clear cause-and-effect relationship. This style comes across as 'distanced and superior' and the doctor is clearly the central actor, with the patient in a subordinate role. By contrast, the relativist and dialogical styles accept greater uncertainty and provide more interaction with the patient and other professionals. Certainly in this case the oncologist, through his narrow focus on causation without thinking of the consequences for his patient and for other practitioners of seeking the genetic test, seems to have acted wholly in the rationalist style. In terms of MacIntyre's 'practices', the standards of excellence to which he aspires are those of scientific medicine, not those of a less-certain personal encounter between practitioner and patient (the 'art' of medicine?).

The various geneticists dealing with Jane and Phyllis would no doubt see themselves as more than simply scientists. The term clinical genetics implies a foot in both camps, and genetic counselling clearly requires a dialogical style. Jane's first encounter was with a person skilled at conveying the very complex interrelationships between genes and occurrence of disease. She seems to have succeeded in conveying the essence of the scientific account of the problem, which is that at the present time there is a lot of uncertainty and that the reliability and sensitivity of current tests are less than ideal. This seems to fit the 'relativist' style of diagnosis described by Widdershoven and Weijts. Patients can find this unsettling and frustrating and one can see how Jane found the greater certainty associated with mastectomy a better relief for her anxiety!

What are we to make of the reactions of the geneticists to Phyllis's refusal to allow her information to be passed on to Jane? Here the values at stake are both humanitarian and scientific. From a scientific perspective such a refusal is irrational and incoherent: why have a test for a genetic mutation solely for your own information when you already know you have cancer? For this reason the geneticist wants to work within a framework in which the test is always sought for family reasons and where the burden of informing relatives (she significantly uses the word 'onus') is carried by the patient. Faced with the anomaly of Phyllis's refusal to divulge the information, the geneticists are willing to resort to various ways of righting the situation, as they see it. 'Hard persuasion' is tried on Phyllis, but to no avail, so then a reconceptualisation is offered: 'Phyllis's test result really belongs to her whole family, not just to her.' (This, however, was not said to Phyllis when her blood was taken.) Finally, the geneticists come out in favour of breaching confidentiality and telling Jane 'in as sensitive a way possible'. (It is unclear what this means, since Phyllis is the one likely to be harmed by the disclosure.) One can see both scientific and moral frustration affecting the geneticists here. Scientifically, restricting such test results to the affected individual is a waste of invaluable information. From a moral or humanitarian perspective, such an insistence on privacy is harmful to Jane and others who may be affected by the information. What then would be a 'virtuous geneticist' approach in such a setting? The practice of clinical genetics does not yet seem to be equipped to answer this question. Are fidelity to the facts and commitment to the best uses of science the excellencies of this practice, or must this scientific dedication be moderated by the commitments acquired through the clinical encounter with the individual tested? The practitioners in this case do not seem to have resolved this tension satisfactorily.

This leaves us with an interesting conundrum with which to conclude this virtue-ethics account of the case. The virtues relevant to human relationships, which illuminated the experiences of Jane and Phyllis and the dilemmas of their GPs, seem somewhat removed from the more intellectual virtues of the science of genetics, influencing the attitudes of the oncologist and geneticists. Are there then two quite separate arenas of virtue, two different worlds, as it were, in which human excellence may be exercised? If so, how can we speak of the 'science of medicine'? Yet do we not separate these worlds at our peril?

REFERENCES

Beauchamp, T. and Childress, J. (1994). *Principles of Biomedical Ethics*, 4th edn. Oxford: OUP.

Bellah, R. (1985). *Habits of the Heart: Individualism and Commitment in America.* Berkeley: University of California Press.

Campbell, A. V. (1984). *The Gospel of Anger.* London: Society for Promoting Christian Knowledge.

  (1998). The Ethics of Care as Virtue Ethics. In M. Evans, ed., *Advances in Bioethics.* London: JAI Press.

Campbell, A. V. and Swift, T. (2002). What does it mean to be a virtuous patient? *Scot J Health Care Chaplains*, **5**(1), 29–35.

Crisp, N. (1996). *How Should One Live? Essays on the Virtues.* Oxford: Clarendon Press.

Gillon, R. (1994). The four principles: a reappraisal. In R. Gillon and A. Lloyd, eds., *Principles of Health Care Ethics.* Chichester: John Wiley, 319–33.

MacIntyre, A. (1985). *After Virtue: A Study in Moral Theory*, 2nd edn. London: Duckworth.

May, W. F. (1983). *The Physician's Covenant.* Philadelphia: Westminster Press.

  (1991). *The Patient's Ordeal.* Bloomington: Indiana University Press.

Nussbaum, M. (1988). Non-relative virtues: an Aristotelian approach. In P. A. French, T. E. Uehling and H. K. Wettstein eds., *Ethical Theory, Character, and Virtue.* Notre Dame: University of Notre Dame Press.

Parfit, D. (1984). *Reasons and Persons.* Oxford: Clarendon Press.

Pellegrino, E. and Thomasma, D. C. (1998). *For the Patient's Good: The Restoration of Beneficence in Health Care.* Oxford: OUP.

Simpson, P. (1997). Contemporary virtue ethics and Aristotle. In D. Statman, ed., *Virtue Ethics: A Critical Reader.* Edinburgh: Edinburgh University Press.

Statman, D., ed., (1997). *Virtue Ethics: A Critical Reader* (Introduction). Edinburgh: Edinburgh University Press.

Widdershoven, G. A. M. and Weijts, W. (2002). Diagnostic Styles in Clinical Relationships. In K. W. M. Fulford, D. L. Dickenson and T. H. Murray, eds., *Health Care Ethics and Human Values.* London: Blackwell.

5

Interpretation and dialogue in hermeneutic ethics

Guy Widdershoven

In healthcare practice, patients and their caregivers can sometimes be confronted with complex and difficult problems. The situation confronting Jane and Phyllis in the case described in Chapter 2 is a good example. Should Jane have a mastectomy or not? This is not an easy question for her, or for those around her (her husband, her friends and the various healthcare professionals who are involved). Should Phyllis (be made to) cooperate by providing access to her test results? Although Phyllis is outspoken in her refusal, this does not mean that the professionals agree that the case is closed. Those who find themselves in cases such as this one are often uncertain about how to make sense of the situation in which they find themselves. They come up with solutions at one moment, and have doubts about them the next. The participants often have very different views about what is to be done, depending on their former experiences and background.

One way to approach such problems is to try to do away with ambiguities and to reach an objective impartial view of the situation. With this view, if people are hesitant about what would count as appropriate solutions, this is because they do not yet have enough information about risks and benefits, and have not adequately made up their minds about their preferences. Here, if people have different views of the situation, we need to investigate which view is (more) correct. The underlying idea here is that for each problematic situation there is an ideal solution, which can be found (or at least approximated) by clarifying the relevant facts and values. Feelings of ambiguity and a diversity of views are to be replaced by a clear and unbiased solution.

Hermeneutics is fundamentally opposed to such tempting notions of clarity, objectivity and impartiality. Hermeneutics holds that knowledge is always a matter of interpretation and that all understanding is based upon pre-understandings, which are never totally open to reflection. On this view, feelings of ambiguity and the existence of a variety of perspectives are to be regarded not as a hindrance to our understanding of the situation but as its very precondition. Understanding takes the form of a narrative quest rather

Case Analysis in Clinical Ethics, ed. Richard Ashcroft, Anneke Lucassen, Michael Parker, Marian Verkerk, Guy Widdershoven. Published by Cambridge University Press.
© Cambridge University Press 2005.

than of straight explanation. The fact that people are not sure what to do, and have different views about what is important, should not be seen as problematic but as a positive starting point for further exploration. From this perspective, by contrast with the former, when someone says that (s)he is certain about what is right there is need for suspicion. The moment a perspective is presented as objective and impartial, there is need for critique.

What are the implications for healthcare ethics of taking ambiguity and variety of perspectives seriously? How can one decide what is good if there is no single right solution? Is it not necessary to draw the line at some point, and declare some views or perspectives out of court? Can one really never say that someone is utterly wrong or that some proposition is morally improper? Such issues have been dealt with extensively by hermeneutic philosophers such as Gadamer (1960), Ricoeur (1983) and Habermas (1991). They have defended the view that hermeneutics implies that in practical situations one *can* distinguish between right and wrong, not on the basis of objective criteria but through *practical experience* and on the basis of *communication and deliberation*. They have argued that the hermeneutic approach is a means for moving beyond the opposition between objectivism and relativism (Bernstein 1983).

Important as these theoretical arguments are, it remains to be seen what they actually imply when one aims to develop a hermeneutic ethics relevant for healthcare practice. What can we say about the problems of Jane and Phyllis by focusing upon aspects of ambiguity and differences in perspectives of the participants? What is the use of listening to the stories of those involved if we want to find better ways of dealing with the situation? In order to answer these questions, I will first discuss the notion of *interpretation*, which is central to hermeneutics. I will show that the stories of Jane, Phyllis and the professionals express different ways of interpreting the situation and dealing with ambiguity. Next I will elaborate the hermeneutic view on the role of a *variety of perspectives*. I will argue that the stories of the various people involved show that a confrontation between different perspectives can result in a new and richer point of view but that this is never easily realised. Finally I will explore the question of how a hermeneutic ethics can actually help to improve healthcare practices. I will argue that hermeneutics can raise the moral quality of practice by stimulating the participants to interpret the situation in such a way that ambiguity is taken seriously and by urging them to continue to foster processes of *merging of perspectives*.

Interpretation and ambiguity

According to hermeneutics, human experience is essentially a process of seeking understanding. Human beings *interpret* their situation and try to make sense of it. This is not primarily a conscious achievement but a preconscious process of becoming at home in a situation by responding to it. Understanding is not a matter of 'knowing that' but of 'knowing how'. It is a practical and not a theoretical activity. Gadamer characterises the process of understanding as *play* (Gadamer 1960, 1977). Like a child bouncing a ball, moving it rhythmically and getting immersed in the movement, a person who interprets a situation gets attuned to it and is drawn into it. The experience of being drawn into a rhythmical process is evident if one reads a book or watches a film. The book, or the film, only achieves meaning if one becomes part of it, is being moved by it and forgets oneself. Paradoxically, during such a process of forgetting oneself, one does not lose one's identity, but one feels being oneself present and participating in the situation.

Following Heidegger (1927), Gadamer emphasises that understanding is unavoidably based on *preconceptions*. One can only interpret a situation if one already has some prior understanding of it. In entering a situation, one has expectations about it. Such expectations are based upon prior experiences, as well as notions and conceptions that are part of the language one lives in. Every judgement requires prejudgements which are given with the tradition in which one participates. In order to understand, one has to become acquainted with the tradition. This again is not a matter of conscious appropriation. One comes to know a tradition by being immersed in it, responding to its appeal.

Understanding is not an isolated event. It is part of a process of getting involved in the phenomenon, a process that is there already before one actually turns to it and that goes on after one has turned away from it. One already has some expectations of the book or the film before one actually reads or sees it. Those expectations will be influenced by the things one has heard about it. After finishing reading and seeing, the experience continues, as one remembers it and tells others about it. Here again we see the rhythmical movement of understanding. The cycle of expectation, actual experience and remembrance is itself the movement of life (as Husserl, 1976, makes clear in his analysis of the temporal structure of consciousness).

From a hermeneutic perspective, understanding a situation requires that one is able to make sense of it in the light of one's prior experiences and expectations. One cannot understand what happens if one does not have some frame of reference within which the events can be connected in a sensible way. Yet, hermeneutic understanding also requires that one is *open* to the situation, and sensitive to aspects that do not fit in with one's expectations. Every experience is different to what one expects. It is not a mere confirmation of some general pattern of expectation but an event that presents itself as unique and new. It is precisely this difference between expectations and concrete experiences that makes room for new understanding. The experience of this difference raises questions. As long as every thing happens as expected, one does not learn anything new. In the moment that one's expectations are 'unmet', one is confronted with the limitations of one's pre-understanding and is urged to revise one's opinions. Once the situation is experienced as strange and unexpected, the hermeneutic process itself is made explicit. When natural understanding breaks down, the process of understanding becomes reflexive, in the sense that it becomes clear that one has always started from preconceptions, which can prove to be wrong. At that moment, one comes to realise that one needs a new perspective in order to make sense of the situation, a perspective that by definition must go beyond the frame of reference that one had before (Winograd and Flores 1986).

From a hermeneutic perspective, understanding is based upon stories. Our experience is prepared by stories we hear from others, and it is elaborated in stories in which we try to explain what happened to others. Our life is shaped by the stories that are told about it. In such stories, our experiences, which are at first vague and ambiguous, develop a more prominent form. Stories make explicit the implicit meaning of lived experience. In stories, the pre-narrative structure of life is transformed into a narrative structure (Ricoeur 1983, Widdershoven 1993). By telling stories, we shape the world we live in, giving meaning to our experiences. Such stories are ways of finding meaning in difficult situations. This is essentially a process of grasping for meaning, a search or a quest for understanding (MacIntyre 1981). Stories are therefore characterised by ambiguity. If this ambiguity is repressed, the story does not do justice to the complexity of experience and its capacity of meaning-making is impoverished (Frank 1995).

From a hermeneutic point of view, it is important to focus upon the stories that the participants in a case tell. What experiences come to the fore in the stories of Jane, Phyllis and the professionals involved? What are the issues they grapple with? How do they try to come to an understanding of the situation? How do they deal with ambiguity?

Interpretation and ambiguity in the case of Jane and Phyllis

The story of Jane expresses her anxiety about a possible genetic predisposition for breast cancer. It also reveals that this anxiety is part of Jane's family history. Jane recalls her mother's illness, as well as that of her grandmother. She identifies with them, and this heightens her fear of being predisposed to cancer. Once Jane approaches the age at which her mother became ill, the worry about cancer seems to become more meaningful for her. Jane describes how she tries to understand her situation and find a way of dealing with it through visits to her GP, the genetic specialist and the support group. It is easy for Jane to understand her GP and the members in the support group. She feels at ease with their suggestions and is inclined to act accordingly. They fit in with her own views and can be integrated neatly into her story. Jane finds it much more difficult to understand the specialist. The procedure of filling in the family history and the genetic information provided at the first interview evidently do not fit in with Jane's preconceptions (neither intellectually nor emotionally). As a consequence of this, Jane finds it hard to see what the geneticist means. She does not really understand why she needs Phyllis's help. Given that Phyllis is little inclined to cooperate with her family, Jane quickly gives up trying to convince her. The relationship between Jane and the geneticist, and that between Jane and Phyllis are both ambiguous. On the one hand, Jane understands that she needs them to solve her problem better, on the other hand she does not understand in what way she needs their support, and is not able to handle breakdowns in the communication. Thus, the story of Jane expresses a hermeneutic experience: she wants to understand and come to terms with the perspective of others (the geneticist and her aunt) but encounters difficulties in achieving this.

The story of Phyllis is much more straightforward than Jane's. Phyllis feels betrayed, both by her illness and by the people around her. Her relatives are ungrateful and the medical staff are not really interested in her. Her conclusions are firm: she does not feel obliged to do anything, given that no one has ever done anything for her. It seems as though the story is clear, and Phyllis understands her situation quite well. Yet this conclusion is somewhat premature. Can we really say that Phyllis understands the situation because she expresses her views so firmly? In the first place, one may doubt whether Phyllis's judgement of others is really adequate. Is her view that nobody ever was interested in her totally convincing? Phyllis seems to have interpreted Jane's visit as yet another example of her family wanting to make use of her. Jane just needs her for making the genetic test possible. This fits in with Phyllis's preconceptions regarding her family. But this interpretation is, in a way, too easy for it to do real justice to Jane. We hear from Jane that she does not regard Aunt Phyllis as simply a means to get genetic information. She expresses certain worries about Aunt Phyllis's physical and mental well-being. Even if these worries do not result in concrete actions (and thus are not easily recognisable for Phyllis), they show that Jane sees Aunt Phyllis as more than a just means to reach her own goals. In the second place, her understanding of the situation does not help Phyllis much to find ways of dealing with it in such a way that she herself feels happy. It is precisely because Phyllis is sure that everybody is being unfair to her that she has no way to relate to others in a more open and more rewarding way. Her pre-understandings are so massive that they do not allow for any breakdown, and thus for learning new ways of envisaging her situation. Because Phyllis's story lacks ambiguity, it does not really help her to understand her own actions and those of others in such a way that she can find new and better ways of living her life.

The story of the GP shows a lot of consideration. The GP is rather hesitant in formulating a point of view, and constantly refers to the views of others. The GP is open to the problems of Jane. Yet it appears that there are few options to benefit her, given that the partner's view, emphasising confidentiality, is presented as convincing. The GP seems to understand Phyllis's point of view and thinks her refusal is reasonable. The objections of the genetics team against using Phyllis's test results secretly are taken into account; the GP does not take a firm position. The story is rather a search for a balanced solution, taking into account all kinds of arguments. In the end, the notion of confidentiality prevails. This notion is strengthened by reference to the professional code. The discussion seems to be closed although certain questions remain unaddressed. The GP's style of reasoning resembles Jane's in some respects, in that it is open to the perspectives of others. Contrary to Jane, however, the GP does not show any difficulty in understanding other points of view. Whereas Jane struggles in order to understand the geneticist and shows a certain discontent about the outcome of her visit to Phyllis, the GP seems satisfied with the course of events. Whereas Jane in the end still seems uncertain about the right solution, the GP is content with the policy of putting confidentiality first. Subtle as the considerations may be, the story in the end does not express any feelings of ambiguity, and the conclusion does not leave much room for further deliberation.

The story of the oncologist is straightforward. The possibility of benefiting Jane is in the end the guiding principle. The oncologist feels responsible for the patient, and from this concludes that information that may help to specify treatment conditions is of the utmost importance. The preconceptions behind this view appear to be rather rigid. The oncologist equates helping the patient with maximising information about treatment conditions and neglects the fact that patients can sometimes be better helped by other means (for instance, by taking time to discuss the consequences of such information for the patient and the family before deciding to do the test). It seems that for the oncologist other views, based upon other preconceptions, are in the end not relevant. Just as in the story of Phyllis, the story of the oncologist shows little room for ambiguity and once again, one may question whether such a story is tenable and whether it is helpful in finding ways to deal with the situation. Does the story do justice to the views of other parties, such as Phyllis and the geneticist? Does it solve the problems? At first sight the message is clear, and the preferred course of action easily identified. But what is to be done if other parties do not go along with this? Given the certainty with which the solution is presented, one seems to have no other choice but to reject other views ('at the end of the day' they are 'not practical or feasible'). How is one to prevent this from resulting in a clash of powers? And if such a clash were to occur, how would one enforce one's view on the others? The oncologist is not the central figure in the decision about whether or not to use information about Phyllis in favour of helping Jane. Clear as the preferences may be, it may be doubted if they will have much bearing on the further course of events.

The story of the geneticist is at first rather technical. It focuses on the need for a diagnostic-test result in order to perform a reliable prognostic test. Given that the geneticist already has the results of a diagnostic test (in Phyllis), the problem is whether this might be used against Phyllis's wishes. The geneticist is unsure about this. Simply taking Phyllis's refusal for granted does not seem the best course. Persuading Phyllis is no option as all attempts appear to be in vain. The geneticist thinks that the view that Phyllis's test results are her own is not correct. This is formulated in a tentative way: 'I feel that in these situations, Phyllis's test result really belongs to her whole family, not just to her.' Because this is not presented as an overarching principle, it does not lead to a strict conclusion. The geneticist does not state that Phyllis's test result can be used right away. This means that the ambiguity of the situation is presented in the geneticist's story. The conclusion is not that Phyllis's view can be dismissed as irrelevant. Her view matters, but it can and should be criticised. According to the geneticist, Phyllis is in a way irresponsible in withholding the information. By describing the situation in such a way, the problem is no longer interpreted in terms of deontological rules (as the GP does when referring to the professional code) nor in terms of maximising medical possibilities (as the oncologist does) but in terms of mutual responsibilities in concrete relationships. This implies a focus on context and historicity rather than on general rules or principles. The geneticist proposes a procedure to prevent irresponsible behaviour in future cases by making an agreement to the use of results for family members a precondition for testing. It can be doubted whether this proposal does justice to the ambiguity of the situation. It is not clear whether the suggested procedure makes people who want to be tested more aware of their responsibility towards family members. The procedure might actually lead to less discussion about the consequences for other family members. The idea that people who take a test should also take up responsibility towards their relatives might not be promoted by just demanding consent at the outset. Finally, a solution to the present case is formulated. The preferred line of action in the end seems to be to tell Jane about Phyllis's result, albeit 'in a sensitive way'. Only to use the result and not to tell Jane about it would mean that she would guess the source of information anyway. Again one may question whether this solution is totally adequate. In the proposed line of action, the issue of family responsibility is not addressed at all. The fact that the geneticist in a sense takes over Phyllis's responsibility is not made explicit. What telling Jane about Phyllis's result might mean for the relation between the two (for example for Jane's responsibility towards Phyllis) is not discussed. If responsibility is a key issue in such matters, the proposed solution should enable further reflection on such matters rather than closing the discussion.

The stories of Jane, Phyllis, the GP, the oncologist and the geneticist can be seen as different ways of interpreting the situation and finding means to deal with it. In the stories of Jane and the geneticist, the ambiguity of the situation is clearly expressed. Their stories explicitly take the form of a quest, emphasising the complexity of the problem and the need for deliberation. When it comes to formulating solutions, however, the ambiguity tends to get lost. Jane seems to expect the mastectomy to solve all her problems. The geneticist formulates an intake procedure, suggesting that this will prevent problems with confidentiality among family members in the future. The story of the GP takes into account a lot of different considerations. Yet the situation is not really experienced as perplexing. In the end, the discussion is closed by a reference to the professional code. The stories of Phyllis and the oncologist leave little room for complexity and ambiguity. Their arguments are straightforward and their conclusions are strict. From within a hermeneutic perspective, the very clarity of the stories and the proposed solutions may raise doubts about their adequacy. Is this all there is to say, and will the proposed line of action really solve all the problems? But if stating firm and well-grounded conclusions is not the way to deal with problematic situations, then how are we to go about it? How can we find solutions doing justice to the ambiguity of the situation? The hermeneutic answer is to continue the process of searching for meaning rather than closing it; to elaborate stories rather than ending them with conclusions; and to stimulate interaction between stories rather than declaring the interpretations of others irrelevant. One should not focus on one story but make use of the variety of perspectives presented in the stories of all those concerned. In order to make clear what this entails, let us now turn to the hermeneutic notion of the broadening of perspectives and fusion of horizons.

Varying perspectives and fusing horizons

According to hermeneutics, every interpretation requires a perspective. People interpret any given situation on the basis of certain preconceptions. This implies that interpretations of the same situation can be different. Depending on one's preconceptions, one will be inclined to highlight certain aspects of a situation and put others to the margin. One always sees the situation *as* something (Wittgenstein 1957). This means that one does not see it as something else and does not interpret it as it might be interpreted from another perspective. These differences in perspective are evident in the stories of Jane, Phyllis and the healthcare professionals involved in the case. Jane, in asking Phyllis for her cooperation, did not anticipate the blunt refusal. If she had done so, she would not have visited her aunt in the first place. The GP, the oncologist and the geneticist interpret the ethical issues in different ways and come up with solutions that in many respects are opposed to one another. The GP thinks it is natural to abstain from using test information from Phyllis in order to help Jane, but the oncologist tends to approach the issue from the opposite side. Although the geneticist in the end comes to the same conclusion as the GP, the arguments are different and they are based upon different presuppositions.

From a hermeneutic point of view, a variety of perspectives is not only inevitable, it is also *productive*. If there were always only one interpretation, one would never be able to learn something new. If one can see a situation in a variety of different ways, one can develop one's interpretation further. The meaning of a situation is not given – it is itself the product of the history of interpretation (Gadamer 1960). The meaning of a book or film changes when it is reviewed by new critics. Commentaries on works of art do more than to bring hidden meaning to the front; they create new meaning. This is expressed very clearly by Proust in *In Search of Lost Time*, recounting a performance of La Berma. Proust describes how the meaning of the performance was influenced by the expectations of the narrator, to such a degree that the narrator was actually a little disappointed when he heard La Berma's singing. Only later, by telling others about the performance, and reading the reviews, was performance turned into a magnificent event. Here we see not only the role of preconceptions in the interpretation of an event (the expectations of the narrator were so high that it became impossible for La Berma to satisfy them) but also the role of commentaries from others in shaping the interpretation and developing a more definite evaluation of the performance. Although this process seems to raise the question of sincerity (is the final evaluation genuine if it is not based on direct experience but on the reactions of others?), one will have to admit that in many situations one cannot avoid adjusting one's views in this way. One only has to remember one's first attempts to read a complex novel or a difficult philosophical treatise to know that following one's first impressions would not have resulted in a favourable judgement but also would have precluded a more thorough acquaintance of the text .

According to hermeneutics, the existence of different perspectives is a precondition for the development of understanding. To understand a situation requires *being open* to new perspectives. When one holds on rigidly to one's own immediate perspective, one is unable to see that the situation might have more aspects and meanings. Being open to other perspectives, however, does not imply embracing them fully and without reservation. One does not really take another point of view seriously if one just accepts it without further investigation. If one is confronted with another perspective, one should not dismiss it right away because it is strange to one's own preconceptions, but neither should one take it over, leaving one's preconceptions behind. Not only is it impossible to discard one's preconceptions so easily, it also would not lead to a more developed interpretation of the situation.

Gadamer defines hermeneutic understanding as a meeting of perspectives, a *fusion of horizons*. He explains this by examining the notion of interpersonal understanding. Gadamer distinguishes three kinds of knowledge of the other (1960: p. 340ff). The first entails an explanation of the other's behaviour by applying knowledge of human nature. This is not interpersonal understanding in the strict sense of the term, since the other is seen as an object. The second comes to know the other in his or her uniqueness. In this case one claims to be able to understand the other exactly as he is. If one knows in this way, one steps out of one's own perspective and completely enters that of the other. The third kind of understanding of the other is to be really open to what the other has to say. This means that one does not put oneself directly in the place of the other but is prepared to hear what the other has to say and to acknowledge that it may be necessary to change one's own views about the matter. Gadamer (1960: 343) explains this third, specifically hermeneutic, kind of understanding of the other thus: 'When two people understand one another, this does not mean that one "understands" the other in such a way that he sees the other from above, and thus oversees him ("überschaut"). Likewise, to "hear someone and respond to him" ("auf jemanden hören") does not mean to execute blindly what the other wants. A person who acts in such a way is called slavish ("hörig"). Openness towards the other entails the recognition that I myself will have to accept things that are against me, even if no one else pushes me to do so.' According to Gadamer, the third form of understanding requires a *dialogue*. In dialogue both of the participants change. 'To reach an understanding in a dialogue is not merely a matter of asserting one's own point of view, but a change into a communion in which one does not remain what one was' (p. 379). Two points should be added. In the first place, this process of understanding through dialogue is not necessarily (nor even primarily) an intellectual process. Understanding is not based upon a conscious process of looking for points of agreement but upon a preconscious engagement into a common movement. In the second place, the mutuality reached is never a total union; in a dialogue, a common point of view may be reached, but this is always partial (since the perspectives of the participants will never fully overlap) and is in danger of breakdown.

In order to come to a new understanding of the situation and to learn from the perspectives of others, one has to be prepared to listen to them and to attempt to make sense of their way of interpreting what is at stake. One should not dismiss their views as irrelevant but try to engage in a dialogue and find new common ground. This is not easy since one has to be open to the possibility that strange interpretations may in the end be equally or even more important than familiar ones. Is such openness feasible, given the stories of Jane, Phyllis and the healthcare professionals, and what might it amount to if one wants to find a solution for the problematic situation they are involved in?

Perspectives and horizons in the story of Jane and Phyllis

The story of Jane shows at various points that her understanding of the situation is developed by a confrontation with the stories of others and perspectives implied in them. At first her feelings of anxiety almost seem to paralyse her. The visit to the GP makes her view her situation differently and requires her to find a way of dealing with it more adequately. The GP gives her a feeling of control over her own body, so that it is no longer totally alien to her. This can be regarded as a sort of reconciliation with the body, which from a naturally given ally had turned into a strange and potentially hostile other. The need for readjusting one's relation with one's body is put forward in many descriptions of the situation of people who become seriously ill. By taking up the GP's perspective on how to perform preventive actions, Jane is able to see her own body not merely as strange but also as manageable. The fear for the illness is not dismissed but changed into a preventive practice of regularly having mammograms and performing self-examinations. The GP also refers Jane to the genetic specialist. Here again she is confronted with a new perspective. She has to fill in a questionnaire and make sense of complicated information about genetic inheritance. Again, issues that were formerly not relevant are being presented as important for her situation and future. Unlike the meeting with the GP, the confrontation with the perspective of the geneticist does not go smoothly. Jane is not very well able to integrate the point of view of the specialist into her own perspective. The merging of horizons appears to be difficult, both because of the large differences at the start and because the specialist seems to be less able to present her point of view than the GP. Consequently, Jane's perspective is not changed as thoroughly as one might have wanted. The third confrontation with another perspective takes place when Jane visits Phyllis. This interaction is not exactly a hermeneutic dialogue. Jane describes Phyllis as 'a grumpy thing'. Such a description is an example of Gadamer's first kind of knowledge of the other: it is a general characterization, not an understanding of Phyllis's individuality. Hence, Jane learns nothing new about her situation from this meeting. The meeting with other patients in the support group described at the end of the story resembles the visit to the GP. Jane learns that she can actively take her fate in hand by having a mastectomy. Jane is well able to understand this and is inclined to act conformingly. In conclusion, Jane's perspective seems to be enlarged most by her meetings with the GP and the support group. Unfortunately her meetings with the geneticist and her aunt, which might be regarded as more crucial in the process of finding the right way of dealing with the problems around her genetic history, are far less productive. Therefore Jane's understanding of her situation is in the end rather confused. She clearly does not know what is best for her to do.

In Phyllis's story we hardly see any opening of horizon. Phyllis is convinced that everybody is against her. Whatever experience she has, it always tends to confirm her views rather than raise doubts about them. She is disappointed in her family as well as in the medical professionals she meets. Consequently she is not at all inclined to listen to them. If somebody asks her something, she is suspicious and suspects a hidden agenda. Phyllis's attitude towards others is one of making generalisations. She presents an example of the first kind of interpersonal understanding distinguished by Gadamer. The result is that Phyllis becomes stuck in her own perspective. The story is iterative. Does this mean that there are no possibilities at all for Phyllis to change her views? That conclusion seems to be too quick. Her disappointment makes her not very willing to accept that other people might be interested in her. Yet the same disappointment also makes her feel that she misses the understanding of others. Although her experiences with her family and with healthcare professionals have not been very rewarding, she also expresses a need for their attention. If people (either family members or medical professionals) were able to break through her defences, she might actually be able to open up and broaden her perspective.

The story of the GP shows a specific way of interacting with others. The GP tends to listen to the views of others in a sympathetic way, and to go along with much of what others bring up. At the practice meeting, there is easy agreement with the partner's claim that confidentiality should not be broken. Phyllis's reaction is presented as reasonable. The objections of the genetics team against 'fudging' are not being questioned. The attitude of the GP seems to be in line with Gadamer's second kind of understanding of the other: taking over the perspective of the other without questioning it. The GP is not only open but perhaps too open. The result is that the reader does not get a clear view of what the GP has actually learned from the discussions being reported. The GP assimilates other perspectives without showing much commitment to any of them. The conclusion that respecting confidentiality is in the end the most important issue does not seem to be the GP's own personal point of view. In a way, the GP evades personal engagement by referring to the professional code. Moreover, the professional code is regarded as a clear set of rules. As is the case with the perspectives of other people, the GP takes over the code without even wondering in what sense the rules might actually be applied in the concrete situation. This precludes a hermeneutic attitude, which takes into account that rules always have to be applied, which itself requires an interpretation, as is evident in the case of laws, which acquire their meaning in the process of jurisprudence (Gadamer 1960).

The oncologist reports several interactions in which perspectives of others are experienced. These interactions are not with patients (who apparently do not count as persons presenting potentially relevant views in the story of the oncologist) but with colleagues, namely the geneticists. The oncologist learns certain facts from the geneticists, broadening the oncologist's cognitive framework. Yet in normative matters the perspective of the geneticists remains completely strange to the oncologist. Discussions with patients about their responsibilities towards family members are irrelevant for the oncologist, and moreover harmful if they obstruct the use of genetic information for decisions about treatment. Whereas the oncologist is open to other perspectives (those of his colleagues) in cognitive affairs, the normative domain is left out of the discussion. Yet this unwillingness to take seriously the normative perspective of the geneticists also diminishes the possibility to actually enter into a dialogue with them and convince them that they are wrong. It is hard to envisage a discussion between the oncologist and the geneticists resulting in a change of policy of the latter.

The story of the geneticist focuses on confrontations between the perspectives of the genetics team and those of the two clients, Phyllis and Jane. Much emphasis is placed on the differences between the team's views and those of Phyllis. The team is not prepared to accept Phyllis's refusal as definitive – they keep trying to convince her otherwise. In the end, the geneticist concludes that Phyllis is wrong in considering her test results as only belonging to her. By formulating the view that test results are not strictly individual, and holding on to it against the views of others (such as Phyllis), the geneticist appears willing to defend a specific position. In doing so the geneticist does not declare Phyllis's perspective irrelevant. The constant urge to try to convince Phyllis that she should change her mind shows that the geneticist thinks it is possible to bring about a broadening of Phyllis's perspective.

The idea that a merger of perspectives is to be strived for shows a hermeneutic attitude. The way in which the geneticist deals with Jane's perspective is similar: Jane's decision to have a mastectomy is not simply accepted and her conclusions are regarded as unwarranted. Again the focus is on trying to convince the other party. The geneticist aims at a broadening of the perspective of Jane. Compared to the GP, the geneticist is much more inclined to take a position and defend a view. Compared to the oncologist, the geneticist is more eager to actually enter into a debate with people who have a different perspective in order to try to make them broaden their view. The geneticist seems to be prepared to enter into a hermeneutic dialogue with the clients, aiming at a fusion of horizons. Such a dialogue, however, also presupposes a willingness to give up one's own position, should the arguments of the other prove to be stronger. One might wonder whether the geneticist is actually prepared to admit that Phyllis might be right in refusing access to her genetic information, or that Jane might be right in deciding on a mastectomy. As mentioned before, the strict intake procedure proposed by the geneticist is in this respect doubtful.

The stories of Jane, Phyllis, the GP, the oncologist and the geneticist make clear that people's views can be broadened if they are confronted with other perspectives. Jane comes to see her situation differently by visiting her GP and by talking to other patients in the support group. The GP changes his views as he hears other opinions. The oncologist enlarges his cognitive perspective by meeting geneticists. However, the stories also show that a merger of perspectives is not always feasible. The perspectives of Jane and Phyllis do not coincide nor meet that of the geneticist. The normative view of the oncologist is not open for interaction with that of the geneticist. The stories finally make us see that a productive merger of perspectives can only come about if one is prepared to be open to the views of others without simply giving up one's own views. The GP seems to be much too inclined to go along with others. Phyllis and the oncologist seem to regard their own views as definitive.

By looking at the way in which the stories interpret the situation and by focusing on the interactions between various perspectives, it has been possible to establish the problematic features of the situation, and also to give some suggestions for improvement. Is it possible to develop this into a more explicit and systematic view on dealing with ethical problems from a hermeneutic point of view? What would this imply for the case of Jane and Phyllis?

Fostering interpretation and sustaining dialogue

From a hermeneutic perspective, dealing with ethical issues in healthcare practice requires interpretation and dialogue. People have to make sense of their situation in order to be able to live in it. They can only do this if they communicate with others, and thereby find new ways of looking at their life by incorporating other perspectives. Interpretation is a process that is already taking place, before any conscious decision is made. People always seek to make sense of the situation they find themselves in. Yet processes of interpretation can become stuck, especially when they become rigid and are no longer open to ambiguity. As with interpretation, communication flows along by itself. People find themselves relating to one another, responding before the questions are clear. But processes of communication can also be obstructed. They can result in circular movements that do not give rise to new perspectives. People can be trapped in their own perspective, no longer able nor prepared to consider other points of view as potentially valid.

The task of hermeneutic ethics is to help people to continue and to improve the process of interpretation. One way to do this is to draw attention to the complexity of the situation. Hermeneutic ethics is critical of all attempts to frame the problem in terms of strictly defined principles and to solve it through abstract procedures. Hermeneutics underlines the fact that ethical problems in healthcare are always both *complex* and *concrete* (Leder 1994). One should investigate what the situation means for those who are actually involved in it. How do they define the issue? What solutions do they envisage? What problems do they encounter? Hermeneutics is sceptical about interpretations that are general and ahistoric. In trying to make sense of a situation, one should be aware of its intricacy and of its historical and contextual background. In the area of genetics this means that there are no universal rules and principles guiding moral practice. As genetics is a developing practice, new problems occur and new solutions will have to be invented. From a hermeneutic perspective, every case is unique. What is good in one case might be not good in another. Hermeneutics urges participants in a practice to be open to the contextuality and contingency of the situation. It invites people to interpret their situation not within a fixed and rigid set of principles, but by being flexible and open to new possibilities.

Hermeneutic ethics can foster the process of interpretation by actively contributing to it. By introducing a new view on a case, the participants can be provoked to see it differently. Hermeneutic ethics can contribute to the process of interpretation by acting as a *critic*, commenting upon the performance of the participants in the case. This can help the participants to tell new stories about their situation by providing new interpretations, in the same way that the critics in Proust helped the narrator to interpret La Berma's performance differently. An example of this is the analysis above, of the process of interpretation in the various stories. The analysis brought to the fore that the stories of Jane and of the geneticist take the form of a quest, and in that respect can be seen as hermeneutic endeavours. The stories of Phyllis and of the oncologist, on the other hand, are rigid and have little room for ambiguity. The story of the GP is not fixed but neither is it a good example of hermeneutic openness. It is in a way too flexible to be convincing and in the end puts too much trust in the professional code. From this analysis we may conclude that the stories of Jane and of the geneticist deserve further close attention. Their stories are interesting not because they contain the right solutions but because they show hermeneutic work. Hermeneutic ethics can sustain such interpretive work in several ways. One way is to clarify the preconditions for interpretative activities. Another is to elaborate the concepts introduced by people involved in a practice and relate them to philosophical traditions. Both activities imply the introduction of theory.

As an example of the relevance of hermeneutics in *clarifying preconditions* of interpretation, let us have a closer look at the story of Jane. This story makes clear that in order to understand her situation, Jane has to find a new way of handling her body. The advice of the GP is meaningful because it contains actions that make sense to Jane, such as examining her breasts herself. This not only involves rationally valid procedures, it also implies getting a new grip on one's body. Jane's story captures the idea that in order to be able to interpret a situation in which one loses trust in one's body, one needs to find new ways of relating to one's body. One needs new rituals, such as examining one's breasts. The suggestions of the GP are meaningful to Jane because they provide her with a script which enables her to regain trust in her body. Such scripts appear to be missing in the suggestions of the geneticist. Jane does not know how to integrate the latter into her daily life. Although the issues brought up by the geneticist might be scientifically more adequate, for Jane the suggestions of the GP appear to be more meaningful. One thing that may be concluded from this is that the geneticist should pay more attention to what actually fits in with Jane's way of handling her situation and relating to her body. In order to help Jane to come to terms with her situation, one should provide her with options that make sense to her. Jane's story can be read as a plea for taking into account issues of embodiment in genetic counselling. The consequences of this may be examined further by relating Jane's experience to theoretical work about, for instance, rituals and scripts (Akrich 1992) or to theories of autonomy, which focus upon providing people with choices that actually have meaning for them (Agich 1993).

Hermeneutics might also help to *elaborate concepts* introduced in stories of practitioners. In order to illustrate this, let us have a closer look at the story of the geneticist. The geneticist argues that Phyllis is wrong to consider her test results as something private. In this argument, the notion of family is brought up. The geneticist considers family relations in a sense more important than individual autonomy, at least for the problem under consideration. The concept of family and its relevance for the issue at hand can be further investigated by introducing theories that specifically analyse such matters. The story of the geneticist might, for instance, be connected to theories in the area of care ethics, focusing on relational autonomy (Mackenzie and Stoljar 2000). In her argument, the geneticist implicitly uses a notion of responsibility, when criticising Phyllis for withholding information. This critique can be related to philosophical work on responsibility (Tronto 1993, Walker 1998). This might strengthen the conclusions of the geneticist but it might also show that they need to be specified or modified. Conversely the connection between stories and theories might also be theoretically productive, in that the application of theoretical concepts and distinctions to practical issues may help to further develop the theories under consideration.

Hermeneutics argues that processes of interpretation are based upon dialogues between perspectives. People make sense of situations in which they find themselves by relating their own perspective to that of others. This process is not directed by the participants consciously. It takes place as soon as people react to one another, ask questions, respond to requests, and thus confront one another with a new point of view. Often this process goes smoothly, and perspectives are merged easily. At other times, perspectives hardly meet, and a fusion of horizons seems unfeasible. In such cases, hermeneutic ethics can contribute by helping the participants to become more open to one another and to actually engage in a dialogue, rather than to remain closed within their own perspective. Hermeneutic ethics can act as a *catalyst*, creating new points of contact and stimulating processes of fusion of horizons through dialogue.

What might this mean in practice? How can the hermeneutic ethicist contribute to the continuation of dialogue? The stories of Jane, Phyllis and the professionals show that at crucial points contact between various perspectives is lacking. One example is the communication between Jane and Phyllis – they are not open to one another. Jane characterises Phyllis as a 'grumpy old thing'; Phyllis interprets Jane's request as another example of abuse. As long as they view one another in this way, Jane and Phyllis will continue to be unable to understand one another and to come to an agreement. What is needed is an intermediary who can serve as an interpreter in the way that Hermes served as an intermediary between gods and humans, an interpreter of the Gods. Where is such an intermediary to be found? In the story of Jane and Phyllis, one might think of Uncle George. He has told Jane where to find Phyllis. This at least shows that he is in contact with both of them. Maybe he is able to understand Jane's situation as well as Phyllis's history and thereby can find a way to make them communicate more openly.

It is not only the interaction between Jane and Phyllis that is problematic; the same holds for those between the geneticist and the clients, Jane as well as Phyllis. Jane has trouble in understanding the information provided by the geneticist. She is not able to fit it into her daily practice. Jane's story shows that the communication between her and the geneticist needs to be improved. It also shows some concrete points deserving attention. One is the time lag between visits. Another is the kind of assignments Jane receives. She is evidently uncomfortable with filling in the family history; she is also unhappy when she is urged to visit Phyllis. In both cases, the geneticist seems not to perceive what such assignments might mean for Jane. From this it may be concluded that the counselling procedure should be reconsidered and brought more in line with clients' expectations and better able to anticipate clients' problems. Phyllis's story shows that she was confronted with strange requests from the geneticists, who appeared to be more interested in her relations than in herself. Again this suggests that communication procedures might need more attention.

The hermeneutic ethicist can make use of the stories of the participants in order to develop concrete suggestions for improvement. This might also entail a better view by the participants of their own role in the dialogue. The hermeneutic ethicist might, for instance, discuss the self-conception of geneticists. Traditionally, genetic counsellors have viewed their activities in terms of *non-directiveness*. Often this is interpreted as providing information without taking any stance and one might wonder whether this does justice to the actual role of the geneticist. In the case of Jane and Phyllis, the geneticist criticises Phyllis's position and implies that Phyllis should reconsider her point of view. This implies that genetic counselling is not just about providing information. It can also entail aspects of interpretation (trying to find out what the client's most fundamental values are) and deliberation (urging the client to critically examine values) (Emanuel and Emanuel 1992). Genetic counselling might entail a more active approach of the client focusing on moral learning on the side of the client (Arras 1990, White 1999).

A third area in which communication is problematic in the case of Jane and Phyllis is in the nature of the relationships between the professionals. The perspectives of the GP, the oncologist and the geneticist do not have much in common and communication among them is mostly absent. The GP refers patients to the genetics centre without apparent knowledge of what goes on there. The oncologist does not understand the geneticist's concern for family relationships. The discrepancies between the perspectives not only hinder mutual understanding between the professionals, they also make things confusing for the clients. More communication between professionals involved with genetic testing therefore seems to be needed, not only in the interests of the professionals themselves but also in that of the clients. In the area of genetics discussion between professionals might be improved, not only concerning cognitive problems but also concerning moral issues. Hermeneutic ethics can play a role in organising communication and debate between various professionals on the ethical issues involved in dealing with genetic information.

To summarise, the task of hermeneutic ethics is to foster interpretation and to sustain dialogue between all the participants. This precludes the taking of a neutral position. The hermeneutic ethicist can only comment upon the stories of the participants if he or she has a perspective on him- or herself. Stimulating dialogue requires that one intervenes in the debate. Just as the participants tell their story in order to find solutions to the problematic situation, so the hermeneutic ethicist interprets these stories in order to help develop new solutions. The hermeneutic activity of the ethicist is in this sense no different from the hermeneutic endeavours of those who are involved in the practice under consideration.

REFERENCES

Agich, G. J. (1993). *Autonomy and Long-Term Care*. Oxford: Oxford University Press.

Akrich, M. (1992). The de-scription of technical objects. In W. Bijker and J. Law, eds., *Shaping Technology/Building Society*. Cambridge, Mass: MIT Press, 205–24.

Arras, J. D. (1990). Aids and reproductive decisions having children in fear and trembling. *Milbank Quarterly*, **68**, 353–82.

Bernstein, R. J. (1983). *Beyond Objectivism and Relativism*. Oxford: Oxford University Press.

Emanuel, E. J. and Emanuel, L. L. (1992). Four models of the physician–patient relationship. *JAMA*, **267**, 2221–6.

Frank, A. W. (1995). *The Wounded Storyteller*. Chicago: Chicago University Press.

Gadamer, H.-G. (1960). *Wahrheit und Methode*. Tübingen: Mohr.

(1977). *Die Aktualität des Schönen*. Stuttgart: Reclam.

Habermas, J. (1991). *Erläuterungen zur Diskursethik*. Frankfurt am Main: Suhrkamp.

Heidegger, M. (1927). *Sein und Zeit*. Tübingen: Max Niemeyer Verlag.

Husserl, E. (1976). *Ideen zu einer reinen Phanomenologie und phanomenologischen Philosophie*. Erstes Buch. The Hague: Martinus Nijhoff.

Leder, D. (1994). Toward a hermeneutical bioethics. In E. Dubose, R. Hamel and L. O'Connell, eds., *A Matter of Principles?* Valley Forge: Trinity Press International, 240–59.

MacIntyre, A. (1981). *After Virtue*. London: Duckworth.

Mackenzie, C. and Stoljar, N. (2000). *Relational Autonomy*. Oxford: Oxford University Press.

Ricoeur, P. (1983). *Temps et récit, I*. Paris: Editions du Seuil.

Tronto, J. C. (1993). *Moral Boundaries: A Political Argument for an Ethic of Care*. New York: Routledge.

Walker, M. U. (1998). *Moral Understandings*. London: Routledge.

White, M. T. (1999). Making responsible choices. An interpretive ethic for genetic decision-making. *Hastings Center Report*, **29**(1), 14–21.

Widdershoven, G. A. M. (1993). The story of life. In A. Lieblich and R. Josselson, eds., *The Narrative Study of Lives. I*. London: Sage, 1–20.

Winograd, T. and Flores, F. (1986). *Understanding Computers and Cognition*. Norwood, New Jersey: Ablex.

Wittgenstein, L. (1957). *Philosophische Untersuchungen*. Frankfurt am Main: Suhrkamp.

6

'Power, corruption and lies': ethics and power

Richard Ashcroft

The standard approach to medical ethical analysis of problematic situations, such as the one concerning Jane, Phyllis and the various medical practitioners in this case, is to identify the 'ethical issues' that the case involves, and then to apply principle- or consequence-based techniques of analysis and arguments to offer some kind of resolution of these issues. Taking this approach, we could, for instance, start by noting the centrality of confidentiality in this narrative. We would seek to analyse the concept of confidentiality in the hope that this would enable us to understand what the limits of the concept are, and to draw inferences about when breach of confidence might be justified or even required, and when alternative principles (such as a duty to minimise preventable harm to others) might be said properly to override an individual's preference that some information about them be held confidentially.

A second feature of the standard approach to medical ethical case analysis is that we are primarily concerned with right action (what should I do?), and in particular right action by a specific actor or set of actors – the medical professionals involved in the situation. (The same goes for nursing ethics and nurses, or counselling ethics and counsellors, for instance).

This approach has been highly productive in both assisting clinicians to deal with ethical and practical problems, and in the intellectual development of medical ethics. However, many commentators have argued that this standard approach is intellectually and sociologically unsatisfactory, since it leaves out of the picture any account of the central role of power relations in establishing the state of affairs under analysis, in constraining the set of options available to the actors, and in defining who has a voice in the given situation. Moreover, it implies that the central moral features of the actors involved are reasonableness, perplexity, incomplete information and, perhaps, moral indeterminacy relating to the balance of competing principles, or the underdetermination of practical requirements by value or principle commitments. To put it another way, it is optimistically assumed that sharing information, opinions and perspectives, thinking hard around different aspects of the problem, and reasonable

Case Analysis in Clinical Ethics, ed. Richard Ashcroft, Anneke Lucassen, Michael Parker, Marian Verkerk, Guy Widdershoven. Published by Cambridge University Press.
© Cambridge University Press 2005.

conversation will provide a way through the problems besetting the identified actors to an outcome that is just, good and consensual.

In the sociological literature on medicine, and in much post-war continental philosophy, we see the lineaments of a much more pessimistic and militant understanding of the nature of problem resolution in medicine and its ethics. Medical problems are taken to involve profound imbalances of power between socially high-status individuals and supplicants in welfare states, or merely economically rational consumers elsewhere. Modern medicine is backed up by scientific practices that constitute a social order based on measurement, calculation and social control, organising people into disease (or future disease) categories for their effective management, surveillance and monitoring. Taken for granted, social worlds of solidarity and mutual support – such as the family – are reorganised in the interests of capitalist production, with the rise of healthcare as a means to the end of efficient industrial production, by replicating the workforce, raising productivity and palliating social unrest. The family later becomes merely a site in which the sexual and reproductive 'labour' of people can be monitored, channelled and regulated. Finally, social life becomes merely a terrain of the definition, organisation and control of 'risk', and the 'citizenry' becomes so conditioned to a discourse of risk management that it cannot effectively step back and analyse how all this happened, how it could be changed and what alternative forms of life could take its place.

In this 'new map of hell', a picture of the social significance of genetic testing and counselling can readily be drawn. Genetic testing draws together a number of strands:

- The practice of individualising risk and the transformation of the good human life into the life of self-surveillance and health optimisation as an individual moral duty.
- The redefinition of the family as a biological category and the evaluation of families on the basis of their set of genetic risk profiles (hence the importance of carrier testing).
- The construction of genetic obligations to others (to disclose information or to pass on, or not, 'good' or 'bad' genes).
- The identification of personal identity with the individual's genome and its 'future diary'.
- The genetic–economic evaluation of individuals in the marketplace (in insurance or employment).
- The role of the doctor as the gatekeeper and evaluator of the option set of individuals, the guide and counsellor to the individual in the face of their future history, and the discrete provider of a panoply of services (at a price) for managing risk.

In this picture, Angus Clarke's famously heretical view that 'non-directive' counselling is impossible becomes not so much a statement of the moral involvement of the clinician in the 'proband's' decision-making, as an indicator of the inextricability of genetic testing and counselling from its social context, which is profoundly shaped by a diverse and perhaps inescapable web of power relations, historical structures and capitalist ideology or 'governmentality'.

The importance of this ebony-black picture of genetics and medicine in capitalist modernity is dialectical. It challenges the self-image of the bioethicist and of the practitioner of healthcare genetics – self-images that could not be further from this alternative image. It is resolutely antipractical: it stimulates 'pessimism of the will' rather than hinting at ways forward. There is a certain pleasure to be taken in elaborating it – rather akin to the pleasure teenagers sometimes take in black metal rock music and in telling their uncomprehending parents that the Earth is heading for a nasty toxic end (and it's all their fault); this is the pleasure of the 'less deceived'. More than this, though, the power of this image is in its ability to evoke a negating response: no, it is not thus; or no, it is thus, but there must be a way out; no it is thus, and we may not change it, but good will and honest struggle will sustain hope. Most of all, the challenge of this picture is to take it on its own terms, to take up the challenge of identifying and characterising the power relations suppressed from the medical ethicist's image of problem-solving as practical reasonableness and liberal consensus, and to think normatively about the use of power and, perhaps, about tactics of resistance. The doctor may be a powerful agent; what ought he or she in good faith do with that power? The patient may be less powerful; what can we do about that?

In the remainder of this chapter, I will discuss three main theories of power and illustrate how they capture specific features of Jane's story. I will then discuss what normative conclusions they support in Jane's story.

Power and domination

The central theory of power in social relations is a theory of power as a scarce resource, which certain agents or institutions have in excess of other agents, and which permits the more powerful agents to control, coerce or induce the less powerful agents to do their bidding. On this theory, doctors are typically more powerful than their patients, and patients are largely compelled to do as their doctors wish. Power structures in this theory are not necessarily rigid or robust, and they may to some extent be invisible or concealed from the parties whose relationships they structure. In modern societies where authorities are generally expected to give reasons for their decisions, and the use of force is permissible only within relatively narrow limits, forms of legitimation take on a special importance. The techniques and tactics of power become diversified to include sophisticated ideological and cultural representations to actors of the grounds and contexts of action, which render particular distributions of power 'natural' or 'rational'. Nevertheless, underlying this ideological representation is a different economy of power that can be explained in various ways, most notably by the relations of production in a capitalist economy (following Marx) or monopoly of the means of forceful coercion (following Weber). The complex relations of 'base and superstructure' entail that most actors will grasp only dimly and intermittently the true nature of the relationships in which they are enmeshed.

This theory of social power is well known, and much of the social theoretic literature of the last 25 years has been devoted to analysing and criticising it. It has a very complex relationship to ethics. At the simplest level, it puts into question the very idea of ethics. Through its critique of the relationship between agents' self-understandings and their true social position and interests, it renders problematic the idea that self-consciously 'ethical' methods of ordering one's actions can authentically engage with the context of those actions. On the one hand, the representation one has of one's situation, the options for change that are available, and the desirability and feasibility of those various options may be fatally compromised by ideological distortions. On the other hand, the possibility of authentically choosing an action that is contrary to one's own interests (in the case of the dominant class) or doing anything genuinely liberatory is put into question by the supraindividual and regulatory nature of the existing power relations, their dominatory force and their conformance to the interests of a particular class. In Adorno's proverb, 'wrong life cannot be lived rightly'.

Yet the theory of social power as domination does leave some scope for ethics, albeit of a 'subaltern' kind. Implicit in the contradiction between the ideological representation of the social order and that order itself lies the possibility for critique of that representation. To the extent that production of a dominant image of society, which covers over the power relations in that society takes continuous work and effort, the possibility of resistance to this work remains open. The image of an order maintained through the continuous production and reproduction of social inequalities contains within itself the Utopian moment, an image of an alternative order, or at least of the possibility of an alternative (even if the form that alternative could take is not clear).

Hence the approach of *Ideologiekritik* implies on the one hand a criticism of ethics as a component part of the dominant ideology, but on the other hand an ethical relation to that ideology and the social order that produces it. This ethical relation calls for agents to engage in a number of critical and revolutionary strategies: deconstruction of the dominant ideology (seeking the implicit contradictions, dramatising or satirising them); constructing Utopian alternatives to mobilise change; and specific strategies of resistance to particular structures or techniques of domination. In philosophy, the principal exponents of this approach are Theodor Adorno, Ernst Bloch, Jean-François Lyotard and Jacques Derrida. The work of Walter Benjamin, Jürgen Habermas and Emmanuel Lévinas have certain methodological affinities with this approach.

There are two obvious kinds of limitations to this theory of power. The first is practical. Under this theory, there are serious epistemological problems created by the theory of ideological distortion for agents wishing to know what their true interests are and what options are both actual and desirable. Moreover, the theory is so 'totalising' that it is far from clear whether there is any scope for private, authentic freedom of action and belief, unconstrained by the structures of power and ideology. There appears to be little room for any metaphysical or moral autonomy, rendering the Kantian questions 'What must I do?' and 'What may I hope?' ill posed and hence unanswerable. Under such conditions, what Peter Sloterdijk calls 'cynical reason', the self-reflexive search for the self-interested motive beneath all utterance, action and institutional form, rapidly replaces Utopian critique. This replacement is possible because of the apparent inextricability of Utopian hope from its ideological representation as self-interested, impractical or available only on the dominant class's terms.

The second criticism is theoretical. The theory of power as domination neglects ways in which power can be constructive or productive, and illegitimately imports a negative evaluation of power. The latter can be explained by understanding that the theory of power of domination begins as a theory of inequality and of limitations on freedom, both of which are (reasonably enough) taken to be bad things; this evaluation then carries over to those agents or structures that are taken to create or constitute such inequality or limitations on freedom. This does little justice to the sophisticated social theories of Marx or Weber, which eschew the narrow moralism this explanatory model implies. However, what their theories do share with this model is a moral critique of the social structures that order the behaviours of both dominators and dominated. This explanatory model in turn derives from a forgetting of the original thesis, which is that power per se is not evil or corrupting, but rather inequality of power, which can lead to domination of the weaker by the stronger.

There are two principal ways out of this theoretical and practical impasse. The first is to construct a theory of productive power, which remedies the practical pessimism and theoretical moralism of the theory of power as domination by showing the ways in which power can be constructive and constitutive of certain freedoms and ways of being. The second is to construct an avowedly moral theory of power, concentrating our focus on the possibility of an ethics of the use of power.

Productive power

The French philosopher–historian Michel Foucault famously argued, in his middle period works from *Discipline and Punish* (1991) to the first volume of his *History of Sexuality* (1998), that social power was constitutive of forms of social life and human practice. For example, in the latter work, he overturned the classical theory that the Victorian middle class was extensively concerned with the repression of sexuality, showing that, to the contrary, it was obsessively interested in investigating, analysing and classifying the phenomenology of sexual desire and practice, thereby creating a whole swathe of new 'perversions' and forms of sexual life, and further inventing whole new classes of individual, for instance, 'the homosexual'. Where formerly there had been only men who had sex with men, now there were 'homosexuals' who had whole sets of norms of behaviour, dress, association, language, and normal and abnormal expressions of their desires. Foucault argues that this reconstitution of society and human nature involved both repression and coercion, domination and control of certain individuals and the creation of new possibilities and styles of existence, permitting a thoroughgoing aesthetics of existence to flourish.

Foucault's work in the earliest phase of this theoretical development tended to concentrate on the way in which the 'iron cage of rationality' (in Weberian terms) imposed itself violently on various kinds of vulnerable social subject – the mad, the sick, prisoners, hermaphrodites, the sexually unusual and so on. It is, however, possible to read his work as showing how many social situations and social groups become safer or more autonomous. For example, Foucault's theory of health and illness shows how the rise of surveillance medicine, the transformation of the body into the site of surgical and laboratory investigation, and the construction of ever finer-grained canons of physical and mental pathology permit at one and the same time the reassignment of certain individuals from the category of the wicked to that of the ill; the extension of lifespan and improvement of the quality of life of many; and the expansion of opportunities for self-expression for many. That said, Foucault explicitly rejects any theory of history, and in particular any theory of history as the history of progress. He underscores the hidden costs paid by the 'winners' in this process, and the very visible costs paid by the losers. His point is that power has multiple effects, constitutive as well as destructive, facilitative as well as coercive; and further that power is not a resource concentrated in the hands of a few but multiply sourced and heterogeneous in its effects.

Foucault's theory is best understood as a kind of phenomenological interpretation of society in combination with a Nietzschean theory of the 'will to power' as creative. He repeatedly refers to the idea of a 'microphysics' or hydrostatics of power, suggesting that we view society as merely the surface phenomenon of a highly dynamic process of forces in precarious balance.

The ethical implications of Foucault's theory of productive power are notoriously difficult to draw out. Some readers take Foucault's theory to underwrite a similar form of ethics as critique to that described when we discussed the theory of power as domination. Others take Foucault's ethic to be frankly Nietzschean, which is to say, essentially a hedonistic amoralism aimed at joyous transcendence of the individual's given situation and the attempt creatively to reshape and dominate that situation. Foucault's own theory of ethics, developed in the last years of his life, notably in the second and third volumes of his *History of Sexuality*, does indeed start from a Nietzschean origin, but draws on a reading of classical ethical literature to construct something nearer in spirit to an ethics of virtue, or the proper use of power in the search for personal excellence. His selection of sexuality as the field for his meditations on ethics is instructive, not because of prurient interest in Foucault's own sexual life but because satisfying and ethically honourable sexual relations require a deep synthesis of emotion, physicality and reflection in the context of a relationship (or series of relationships) with others. Such relationships cannot achieve excellence if constituted purely through a relationship of dominance and submission (although the interplay of moments of each does indeed play a part in sexual desire – the point is that this must be an interplay created by autonomous and equal individuals).

Foucault's theory of power has been widely criticised on a number of grounds. First, he can hardly be said to give a satisfactory definition of power, and his descriptions of the operations of power often give one the sense that his notion of power is so diffuse and heterogeneous that it lacks much explanatory force. Second, his theory of power relations as constitutive of social forms is relatively unproblematic but his account of how power relations create categories of knowledge and conditions of truth, even in the sphere of the biological sciences, seems to precipitate a thoroughgoing cognitive relativism. This reading of his argument can be disputed. Nonetheless, the general thesis that social power is not the sole metaphysical category, and that there are certain natural facts or constraints that it cannot overcome is critical here. A similar criticism can be advanced of the theory of power as domination. Collapse of misfortune or catastrophe into social categories with inequalities of power as the source and as the target of blame is too easy, and neglects some essential features of human existence. Nonetheless, Foucault offers a strategy of interpretation that privileges social agency. In this respect, again, his discussion of homosexuality is important. Homosexuality may or may not have a 'biological' cause yet how the 'trait' is stabilised, what kinds of explanation are sought, what 'treatment', 'punishment' or 'toleration' of it is practised and so on – all of these are socially shaped and mediated, and in that sense the 'natural' or 'unnatural' status of homosexuality as a trait are outcomes of this process, rather than conditions prior to this process.

Power and responsibility

The third theory of power is an expressly normative theory of power. While other normative theories of power, for example that of Spinoza, do exist and have detailed philosophical expositions, they have not been applied to practical problems. The theory of power I will discuss here was developed by US philosopher and professor of family practice Howard Brody. Brody distinguishes three forms of power possessed by the physician that structure the physician's relationship with the patient. He argues that the power of the physician can be used constructively or as a mode of domination (what he winkingly calls 'the dark side of the force'). The main thrust of his book, *The Healer's Power* (1992), is an argument for the sharing of power between doctor and patient, which can best be achieved through the development of a relationship or partnership between doctor and patient. He argues that the ideal context for this to occur is the relationship between patient and family practitioner in primary care.

The three forms of power described by Brody are:

- *Aesculapian power* – the power of diagnosis, prognosis, prescription of treatment, of palliation or of behavioural change, and of communication with the patient, all on the basis of the physician's knowledge, training and experience, which the patient typically does not share.
- *Charismatic power* – the power of personality and personal character to influence the patient.
- *Social or cultural power* – the socially or culturally founded authority of the physician to instruct or require the patient to do certain things, or to respond in a certain way to the communication of certain information.

A good example of the operation of all three types of power in the doctor–patient relationship is a consultation between a doctor and patient who has developed a sexually transmitted disease. The doctor uses his or her Aesculapian power to diagnose the disease and to prescribe appropriate treatment; his or her Charismatic power permits the doctor to cause the patient to adopt safer sexual practices; and his or her Social power authorises the doctor to discuss sexual matters with this patient and to request the patient to change his or her behaviour.

Brody's theory is unsatisfactory from a sociological point of view, in that it does nothing to analyse how the physician's role is constructed, how it arose historically and how it is maintained. As a normative theory it leaves something to be desired because it fails to offer a serious critique of the very idea of the medical authority, and because its theory of how these different dimensions of power are to be employed is somewhat arbitrary and grounded on a tradition of medical practice that Brody criticises but in the end repairs rather than replaces. To the extent that one shares his view of this tradition, this is acceptable, but normatively the problem is that this theory is relatively unspecific about what the criteria of right action are. Rather, his work depends on a series of persuasive case studies, which are very suggestive and illustrative (in the ways the best narrative ethics studies often are) but lack analytic depth.

Notwithstanding these criticisms, Brody's approach is useful. His distinction between the different ways in which the physician possesses a certain power that the patient usually does not does permit us to analyse situations in which the doctor exerts the wrong sort of power towards ends external to the goals of medicine. He also places in the foreground the necessity of reflecting on those goals and on the nature of the 'good doctor'.

Synthetic summary

To review where we are so far: the three theories of medical and social power offer very different accounts of the social context of medical practice; the relationships between doctor and patient; and the possibilities for ethical critique of social power and the ethics of the use of power. From the point of view of social analysis and critique, the theories of power as domination and as productive have more to offer than Brody's theory, while from the normative point of view Brody's and Foucault's theories have more to offer than does the theory of power as domination. In what follows, I draw eclectically on all three theories. From the theory of power as domination, I take the theory of interests and the theory of ethical critique; from the theory of productive power I take the idea of power as constitutive and the idea of the virtuous use of power; from Brody I draw the threefold distinction of the use of medical power as a sketch for the ethics of medical power.

Power in the story of Jane, Phyllis and the doctors

A standard approach to the story of Jane, Phyllis and the doctors would probably start by considering the complex role of medical confidentiality in the story, considering in particular issues of rights to know or not to know information, and a possible duty (either lay or medical or both) to disclose information to a relative who has a vital interest in the information. Secondary issues in the case would be the relationship of the principle of beneficence to the merits of offering a prophylactic mastectomy to Jane, and the arguable professional misconduct of the oncologist in seeking a genetic test as part of the diagnostic work-up without proper prior counselling. The whole story would turn conceptually on questions of risk, its meaning and management.

At first pass, an analysis based on an ethics of power raises similar issues. For instance, the role of the oncologist in the story could be considered emblematic of the excess of medical power and its misuse. Seeking the genetic test in ignorance of the proband's wishes might be thought to show wanton disregard for the ways in which the results of this test could adversely affect the proband's welfare, and indeed the welfare of her relatives. Perhaps this could be explained by the doctor taking an action merely because he could, without proper consideration as to whether he should (is this an appropriate use of his power?) or of the interests of the person to whom the genetic information pertained (is this an illegitimate failure to share power?). This reading of the situation sits naturally in both the Brody theory of medical power conferring responsibility for its proper exercise on the doctor, and in the theory of power as domination. The oncologist's decision is possible because of his social power over Phyllis, and his neglectful failure to consult with her reveals how his representation of the situation dominates the patient's possibility of representing her preferences and shaping the course of actions taken.

Pursuing this line of description, an immanent critique of the ethics of beneficence is possible, apropos of Jane's expressed wish to undergo prophylactic mastectomy. The physician has the power to refuse to perform the mastectomy, overruling Jane's wishes, for the physician has the power to refuse while Jane does not have the power to insist. Hence the physician has the power to define what is or is not beneficent. The situation is not absolutely in the physician's control since the physician has no legal authority to have the operation performed contrary to Jane's wishes. In this situation, part of the efficacy of the physician's power is the power to control the representation of the situation, including, in part, the normative content of that representation (that which ought to be done under the circumstances described). This power is not, as noted, absolute. Yet in another theory of beneficence, the physician might authorise the operation on the grounds that this is primarily a psychological malaise afflicting Jane, and the operation, by satisfying her preferences, will be the most effective way to manage this. While ostensibly this is a sharing of power between Jane and her doctor, the definition of the situation remains under the physician's control, and, in a wider sense, the objective good aimed at in this account of beneficence is defined by the wider profession (in that this approach to managing Jane's case receives professional sanction, which backs up the doctor's right to respond in this way).

Finally, the physician's power is manifest in the power the physician has to reveal clinical information about Phyllis to Jane, overriding Phyllis's express wishes. In part this depends on some merely contingent features of this situation (which could reasonably be discussed in terms of moral luck) — it just so happens that the doctor has some information relevant to Jane about Phyllis, which could easily not have come about. Certainly, had the doctor not had this information, she could not have compelled Phyllis to have a genetic test in Jane's interest, anymore than she can compel Phyllis to tell Jane the results of her test. Nonetheless, the doctor could simply decide, with some justification from a lay point of view, to tell Jane what she knows. It is questionable whether the doctor would be regarded kindly by the regulatory authority of her profession or the courts for doing so; but if she had reason to believe that Jane would have an operation that was unnecessary or dangerous unless she knew that Phyllis (contrary to fact, and contrary to what we know about the sensitivity and specificity of the test) was 'clear', then the courts and regulators would be much more sympathetic. That is to say, the courts would second the doctor's decision that Jane was at serious risk of harm unless confidentiality were breached.

This account of the ethics of power drawing on the standard ethical representation of the 'issues' in this case is unsatisfactory in a number of ways. First, it pays no attention to the motives of the doctors involved in the case; indeed, to the extent that it does, it imputes rather bad motives (thoughtlessness, arrogance and paternalism, perhaps). Second, this description does little justice to the difficulty of the case, and the emotional stress that is surely induced in all the parties. Moreover, it ignores that in the actors' own accounts of the case, the principal direction of anger is not from Phyllis to the doctor, or from Jane to anyone, but from Phyllis to the rest of her family. The doctor is merely an unhappy and unlucky intruder on two interlocking tales of family tragedy and unhappiness: the tragedy of the family history of early death from cancer and the unhappiness of a family rift. The ethics of power here could equally well focus on the power to heal and reconcile, and the power of Jane and Phyllis to harm each other and 'wound' the healer who crosses their path. Howard Brody reprints Vonda MacIntyre's well-known science fantasy story 'Of Mist, and Grass, and Sand', which dramatises the way the healer can be damaged by his or her power as well as the way that power can itself both wound and heal the patient under the healer's care.

It should be noted, in the context of the theory of power as domination, that it is not an essential part of that theory that the dominant party be an intentional dominator of the dominated parties. The classical Marxist critique of political liberalism's illusions, for example, does not rest on the liberal being in bad faith or of disguised ill intentions. Rather, it rests on the way liberalism's individualism mystifies the social and economic structures that permit bourgeois domination of the working class. Hence 'Lady Bountiful' is to be rejected not because she bears her 'patients' an ill will (although Charles Dickens' accounts of certain kinds of middle-class patronage of the poor, and Nietzsche's theory of pity remain unsurpassed in their diagnosis of forms of this ill will) but rather because she mistakes the way her charity reinforces social and economic dependence.

This debate can go either way. And this is, in itself, an indication of the limits of the Brody and power-as-domination normative theories. While they are powerful diagnostic tools, giving rich and suggestive accounts of what is wrong in the case of Jane and Phyllis, they fail as normative accounts because they lack any internal account of what the ends of action should be. As such, they usefully describe a field of struggle but they do not in fact define well alternatives to this field of struggle, or enable one to pick a side in the struggle defined independently of one's prior commitments. They fail to assist the doctor in her decision-making. What they do contribute, however, is a set of resources for redescription of the situation, and for revealing what the power dynamics are. In this sense, the theory of power as domination, as we noted before, facilitates a certain kind of 'subaltern' stance in ethics – unpicking assumptions, demanding the hearing of suppressed voices and insisting that the relations displayed could be otherwise. With this theory, the existing relations of power are so pervasive and unquestioned that it is an act of liberation merely to 'demand the impossible'. These philosophical guerilla tactics aim at disrupting dominant assumptions as an end in itself, without positing any explicit Utopian alternative. (A philosophical exponent of this style of engagement is the late Gilles Deleuze).

Nevertheless, this style of reasoning fails to satisfy those of us with a more optimistic and constructive temperament. It is possible to consider Brody's inversion of the theory of power of domination (into a theory of the ethics of the right uses of power to help and heal, and of sharing that power rather than holding onto it) as a powerful alternative here. Nonetheless, his account fails as a normative theory in a similar way – it incorporates an external ethic of principles, while failing to offer any critique of its own foundations in pre-existing social power structures and the way these (arguably) fatally distort the principled practice of medicine.

Arguably, therefore, a properly Utopian or constructive theory of power must begin by examining the conditions of possibility of the case in hand. Properly understood, the theory of power as domination is not simply a theory of the impact and phenomenology of domination, as perceived by dominator and dominated. Rather, it is a social theory of the constitution and reproduction of structures of domination. As such, it is very difficult, if not impossible, to work backwards from a case to the relevant social theory, and then forwards again to normative conclusions. The theory and the case clash as particulars do with abstract generalities. Nevertheless, we can proceed in two ways from case to the underlying constitutive structures, in order to trace the sinews of power sustaining the problematic features of the case. One approach is to deconstruct the case narratives, perhaps by Derridean or Bakhtinian method, by seeking to make visible the 'trace' of power in the skein of narrative we have before us. For present purposes, I will not follow this line of analysis, for three reasons. First, methodologically this approach is akin to post-structuralist methods of reading against the grain of the text, which are illustrated and discussed in Chapter 7. Second, as I have indicated, this approach is weak since it depends on a prior or posterior choice of social theory in order to ground its critique – or the disavowal of any such grounding – which tends to make its analyses fragmentary and inconclusive. Third, this approach is normatively underdetermined, as we saw above. The second approach is to build our understanding of this case by explicitly relating the case narrative in realist mode to a constitutive theory of social power, and to place the case in the context of the social knowledge that we possess from other sources.

Again, let us start from the centrality of confidentiality in this case. Confidentiality is a matter of importance in medicine and social life because it is concerned with socially constructed methods of permitting the sharing of certain information with certain parties but not with others. This information is held to be confidential because it is sensitive and secret, which is to say that the confider has good reason to wish for it not to be widely known. As such, it figures in the confider's self-fashioning; confidentiality is a form of management of the boundary between the secret self and public face, between personal private sphere and public currency. It figures in the individual's power to control his or her reputation and credibility, and typically involves what Foucault termed a regime of truth – a system of methods of defining what is real and what is not, how this is verified, monitored and how it is represented as information and distributed through networks of communication. What any society takes to be confidential tends to vary widely, in the way that matters regarded as 'taboo' or 'risky' vary, and the definition and policing of the distinction between the confidential and the non-confidential and control of such information and its transmission play a central role in the self-image of that society and in the metaphysics and ethics of personal identity.

Given this sketch of the social theoretic significance of confidentiality, what can we infer about the special significance of genetic information in this narrative? In the narrative, genetic information is confidential because of its power to predict the future, to define the 'true' nature of kinship, to embody moral relationships of responsibility and autonomy, and to warrant certain rather dramatic courses of action. Further, genetic information calls into operation a special set of professional actions, moral and technical judgements and relationships; for instance, it inserts a certain pragmatics and ethics of risk control, and it mandates a personal self-monitoring ethic and the overarching development of a public-health surveillance of the asymptomatic sick and the worried well. Genetic information on the social theory of genetics implicit in this narrative warrants a certain pharmaceutical and surgical restructuring of a person's life, in response to the individual's recasting of herself as an individual with a certain fate that is to be resisted, averted or otherwise managed.

In other words, the role of the geneticisation of family relationships, the further development of the concept of family history and the reassertion of the demands of 'blood ties' over the historical preferences of individuals to break formerly 'merely contingent and socially constructed' ties of kinship all play their part in the deep structure of this case. The power relations in this situation are subtle and unsuspected, relating to deep social trends of reconstructing the autonomous individual in bioscientific terms, and the assertion of a certain normative structure grounded in nature. None of this is to deny the factual basis of the disease process, the relationship to genetic information, the biological kinship of Jane and Phyllis. A Foucauldian reading of this case points our attention to the *selection* of certain facts and relationships as relevant, and the particular ways in which details are developed and assembled, in the light of broad epistemic and social trends.

What is the normative significance of this rereading of the narrative? As with the previous reading drawing on Brody and the theory of power as domination, the principal normative feature here is the attention to the social production of this situation and the contingencies underpinning this production; in essence to say, this could be otherwise, this representation can be set aside in favour of a different one. In one important sense, this is liberatory on these terms alone. To the extent that Phyllis and Jane deem themselves fated to a certain description of their case (the bad sister and the genetically fated daughter), the several readings suggested here provide resources for the women in question for redescribing their situations in other terms, and to escape the pure inevitability of the dominant narratives of obligation and blame, of fate and destiny. To some extent this also frees the doctor from the sense of obligation to 'do something', in the absence of any external guidance on what that 'something' should be. In the wake of this (dim) moment of liberation, a second follows, which might best be thought of as existentialist vindication of one's narrative as one's own chosen account of one's 'thrown-ness' forward into an uncertain future.

Nonetheless, these are weak and insipid responses to a narrative that is powerful and persuasive (and, in that, testimony to the efficacy of the genetic narrative as socially organising and mobilising in the present order). This is, indeed, a common criticism of Foucault's insistence on the all-pervasiveness of power. The Utopian possibility raised by Foucault is not actually grounded in the freedom to resist or refuse dominant narratives of bioscience in this area, but rather in his aesthetic insistence on the moral significance of creatively refashioning the dominant narrative and one's own situation into an authentically chosen form, in the context of fulfilling relationships of friendship, sexual intimacy and political engagement.

A Romantic note

The German Romantic philosophers (in particular, Friedrich and August Schlegel, Novalis and Friedrich Hölderlin) were fond of claiming that no work of art could ever be more than an unfinished fragment, since the ideal that it presented could always only remain out of reach, imperfectly expressed. This expressed both a certain despair at human finitude and imperfection, and a certain hope that whatever was in hand could be improved upon. This observation may not have been the last word in aesthetics (as if, if true, it could have been!) but it is pertinent to a consideration of ethical agency. We cannot, first of all, trace all the lineaments of power in the case of Jane and Phyllis. For we cannot grasp all the constitutive factors that make the situation, nor can we state with any authority that this description that we do offer is the master description. There are subtle currents we may not perceive and currents we may take to be irrelevant. Much of the power in this situation is focused on defining what is relevant, who has agency and who will have the last word. The German philosopher Axel Honneth draws our attention to one dimension of situations of this kind, which is that they always involve a 'struggle for recognition', both internally to each agent (to grasp what is truly at stake for that agent, without self-deception or false compromise) and between agents. Honneth, unlike his mentor Jürgen Habermas, notes that conditions for free and equal discussion over ends must be fought for and achieved. The tests he offers for resolution are not procedural (as with Habermas) but are instead almost experiential: relations of recognition in differing social spheres are the acceptance by all parties that relations of love (as in warm family relationships rather than erotic/sexual relationships), respect for legal rights and legal personality, or social solidarity obtain. Through Honneth's approach, we could argue that what is at stake is a struggle over the meaning of the family bond, or a counterposition of the family bond and the rights of legal personality to non-coercion and non-interference in seeking one's personal ends. Reflection on this model of 'what's up with Jane and Phyllis' draws our attention to a common feature in discussions of this case, which is unconsciously or unwittingly to take sides and to cast one party or other in the role of the unreasonable, unjust or wicked. This reminds us that as readers of the text (or consultants in the case) we are not 'outside' but involved and that the power relations of the case involve us too. We can respond to this 'interpellation' in various ways: an attractive one is to see our responsibility to the parties as to use a sort of generalised Aesculapian power to heal the social wound before us. Yet we know that is not within our power. We could respond, alternatively, by seeking to unpick and restitch the ways in which the conflicting relations of power (understood as violence or domination) damage or constitute the *emotional* suffering of Jane and Phyllis; it might be, in the end, that the biomedical issue at stake is the occasion of the conflict rather than the conflict itself although this seems to be a one-sided view. Recent writing on violence and subjectivity (in philosophy, Derrida and Levinas, for example; in anthropology, Veena Das and Nancy Scheper-Hughes) might help us with one strand in the tangled skein. Yet none of these strategies would be conclusive, any more than the others canvassed so far. I suggest that Honneth's answer is the best one: we cannot pre-empt the struggle for recognition but we can agree that that is what is at stake in the narratives making up this case, and it may be that the sign of a morally tolerable outcome, however temporary and unstable, would be some restoration of mutual recognition by Jane and Phyllis and the doctors, involving mutual regard and concern, as well as the knowledge that some hurts cannot be removed or covered over. A struggle over rights, a fight to determine whose behaviour is good or bad or irresponsible, can stand for itself but it can also mark a lack of something else – a sense of agency, of being respected and cared for, and a determination to reclaim autonomy in a situation where the demands of others seem to dissolve it away.

Conclusion

My discussion of the differing forms of the ethics of power has illustrated the power of these theories to challenge and redescribe the social relations under-pinning medical ethical problems. I have shown how these theories permit the dramatic redescription of these problems as 'dialectical images', which both permit refusal of the dominant narratives and through their very pessimistic form challenge the agent to break through to identify Utopian moments in the image, and to take up strategies of resistance to taken-for-granted assumptions and patterns of power. However, I have also shown how none of the ethical theories of power can be understood as properly normative, either because they explicitly lack a normative dimension, or because the normative content they invoke is weak or inadequate. I have, I believe, shown that these theories are better understood as preparatory to an ethical understanding of the case, a challenge to lay bare and confront the relations of power underpinning the situation in hand, than as genuine models for ethical analysis and normative recommendation about paths of right action in that situation. Finally, I have suggested that an ethical 'supplement' to this fragmentary and unsatisfactory political deconstruction of the case might be found in seeking a reconstruction of the human relationships over against the dominant medical representation of the nature of the problem. In very practical terms, this approach might tentatively lead us to think that it is the relationship between Jane and Phyllis that is truly at the core of this narrative, rather than their biological kinship or the medical importance of information disclosure or exchange. On that basis, it may be that Jane and Phyllis do decide to exchange medical information. But this would be in the context of a re-established relationship rather than on the basis of what an abstract theory of the obligation to share genetic information in order to manage risk might require, and might indeed authorise the doctor to take over.

SUGGESTED FURTHER READING

Scholarly footnotes are hardly ever on hand in the clinical consulting room, or over the dinner table at home, so I have eschewed them. But the reader might find the following books helpful in following up the themes I have sketched in this chapter.

REFERENCES

Brody, H. (1992). *The Healer's Power*. New Haven: Yale University Press.
Foucault, M. (1991). *Discipline and Punish: The Birth of the Prison*. Harmondsworth: Penguin.
  (1998). *The History of Sexuality. Volume 1: The Will to Knowledge*. Harmondsworth: Penguin.

BIBLIOGRAPHY

Adorno, T. (2000). *Problems of Moral Philosophy*. Cambridge: Polity Press.
Bakhtin, M. M. (1983). *The Dialogic Imagination and Other Essays*. Austin: University of Texas Press.
Benjamin, W. (1999). *Illuminations*. London: Pimlico.
Bernstein, J. (2001). *Disenchantment and Ethics*. Cambridge: Cambridge University Press.
Bloch, E. (2000). *The Spirit of Utopia*. Stanford: Stanford University Press.
Das, V., Kleinman, A., Ramphele, M. and Reynold, P. (2000). *Violence and Subjectivity*. Berkeley: University of California Press.
Deleuze, G. and Guattari, F. (2002). *A Thousand Plateaux*. London: Continuum.
Derrida, J. (1980). Violence and metaphysics: an essay on the thought of Emmanuel Lévinas. In J. Derrida, *Writing and Difference*. Chicago: University of Chicago Press, 79–153.
Foucault, M. (2000). *Power: Essential Works of Foucault* 1954–1984, *Volume 3*, ed. J. D. Faubion. Harmondsworth: Penguin.
Fraser, N. (1990). *Unruly Practices*. Cambridge: Polity Press.
Guha, R. and Spivak, G. C., eds. (1989). *Selected Subaltern Studies*. Oxford: Oxford University Press.
Habermas, J. (1974). *Knowledge and Human Interests*. London: Heinemann Educational.
Latour, B. (1993). Irreductions. In B. Latour, *The Pasteurisation of France, followed by Irreductions*. Cambridge, Mass.: Harvard University Press, 153–236.
Lévinas, E. (1991). *Ethics and Infinity*. Pittsburgh: Duquesne University Press.
Lukes, S. (1975). *Power: A Radical View*. Basingstoke: Macmillan.
Lyotard, J.-F. (1988). *The Differend: Phrases in Dispute*. Manchester: Manchester University Press.
Marx, K. (1975). *Economic and Philosophical Manuscripts of 1844*. In R. Livingstone and G. Benton, eds., *Karl Marx: Early Writings*. Harmondsworth: Penguin.
Nietzsche, F. (1994). *On the Genealogy of Morals*, ed. K. Ansell-Pearson and C. Diethe. Cambridge: Cambridge University Press. [Originally published 1887.]
Scheper-Hughes, N. (1993). *Death Without Weeping: The Violence of Everyday Life in Brazil*. Berkeley: University of California Press.

Sloterdijk, P. (1997). *Critique of Cynical Reason*. Minneapolis: University of Minnesota Press.

Strathern, M. (1992). *After Nature: English Kinship in the Late Twentieth Century*. Cambridge: Cambridge University Press.

Weil, S. (2002). *Oppression and Liberty*. London: Routledge.

7

Reading the genes

Rob Withers

Lost in space: in place of an introduction

I cannot begin at the beginning. Yet children in primary school now learn that every text must have an appropriate beginning. A fairy story opens, comfortingly, 'Once upon a time . . .'. What is missed and not taught is the corollary: the opening sentences and the way in which the writing develops from there (the texture) fashions the kind of text produced. So when I now say that I cannot articulate my philosophical approach at the start of this chapter, I am already shaping the material in a particular style.

I can appreciate why the editors have called for an introduction. They wish me to explain my method. They wish to assist you, Gentle Reader. But I cannot begin there because that is not where I am and I do not see the way ahead with such clarity, yet it must be because it was as 'I would prefer not to'[1] work in this way that I was invited to contribute. This is because of my resistance (the significance of the word in this context should become clearer in the course of this chapter) to use the very model we have all been schooled in. Will I nevertheless satisfy the expectation that in this chapter my writing will exemplify a post-structuralist approach?

Plunging into autobiography, starting from 'somewhere, where we are . . . in a text where we believe we already are' [*'Il faut commencer quelque part où nous sommes . . . quelque part où nous sommes: en un texte déjà où nous croyons être.'* (Derrida 1967)][2], and apparent subjectivity are often taken as markers of something 'post'. Regrettably, however, I shall disappoint even in the editors' modest request to engage with the text before us using a post-structuralist approach because I am uncertain about what might count as doing so. Equally importantly, I am uncertain about what would count as *not* doing so: I was impressed when I once heard Geoffrey Bennington describe 'post-structuralism' as an English word for a collection of originally French thinkers, all of whom violently disagree with one another.[3]

Case Analysis in Clinical Ethics, ed. Richard Ashcroft, Anneke Lucassen, Michael Parker, Marian Verkerk, Guy Widdershoven. Published by Cambridge University Press.
© Cambridge University Press 2005.

Immediately we read the text of Jane and Phyllis autobiographically as a reader who intrudes. We 'take sides', perhaps with Jane in her terrible predicament, and her girls, or with Phyllis who seems to have had the worst of it in her family. Or our initial sympathies lie with Jane but we warm to crabby Aunt Phyllis and begin to suspect that Jane's account of her intentions is misleading. For this is a well-constructed narrative and we are resisting readers. The medical practitioner engaged in thinking ethically (or anyone acting and with a concern for ethics) is, however, pressed by the need to decide or to do something, or to have reflected on why to refrain from doing something. She is orientated around reaching a point of saying 'this is what should be done'. I must recognise that pressing concern for what is to be done. I ought not to leave you stranded, needing to decide on a course of action, while I climb the philosophical foothills. I shall look for signposts and shall finish somewhere. If you are caught up there, trying to come to a decision, I'll be back.

Talk about ethics is open textured and metaphorical. The clearly marked path is a mirage and hence I can only explore from where I find myself, caught in this extended metaphor. (However, I shall possibly mix metaphors, which would be a bad thing: dead ducks may come home to roost.) I shall examine 'the text in hand', searching out the chain of signification. For me the interest of that text, the case study, is that it problematises the nature of information about the body, confidentiality and trust. The dictionary – *not*, that is, any handy little dictionary beloved by students writing essays but the big thick one with long explanations and very small type – may be useful to me in this: I shall look up 'confidential', 'confide', 'private', 'business', 'legislators' and 'charlatans', to see which signifiers it associates with these terms.

There are central issues that I shall visit. I shall begin a recent archaeology of the way in which confidentiality, secrecy and covering up information about the body has come to dominate. This secrecy has led to an eliding of distinctions when talking about trust between patient and physician. Paradoxically, talk of trust has generated less confidence in the physician and reduced willingness on the part of the physician to risk being trusted. Some goods may be lost. I try to destabilise the taken-for-granted assumptions that all information about the body, including genetic information, belongs to the patient and that trusting medics means having confidence in them not to reveal any information to anyone. I try to do this in at least two different ways:

1. By examining how secrecy concerning information about the body has come to be seen as natural as covering up the body, I hope to reveal the concealing technology of disguise here. This is to take seriously Barthes' (1973) account of naturalisation. Genetic information is text, yet we think of it *at one and the same time* as body, which belongs. The text is made into a natural object, part of the body of the patient, to which nothing can be

done without their permission. The discourse of confidentiality founded on trust hides from us the differences between body and text; the discourse signifies a single, common process.

2. I try to learn from one of Foucault's important questions. He asks, what does this kind of discourse consist in 'if not in the endeavour to know how and to what extent it might be possible to think differently instead of legitimating what is already known?' I endeavour to remind us that what has become by a process of naturalisation familiar and everyday is still strange and mysterious. I do this in a shorthand way. That is, not by the clear but long route of using ethnography, rendering the banal anthropologically strange, but by a perhaps less familiar method of drawing attention to the nature of writing about ethics and by investigating its metaphors.

Immediately the practitioner acts, she finds that her decisions are questioned. Unintended consequences become clear, new considerations throw her previous conviction of the rightness of her conclusion into doubt. Suddenly, other possibilities occur to her or are suggested. Pertinent matters that were previously concealed are uncovered. It is discovered that stories that she believed to be accurate had been embroidered, whether knowingly, unknowingly or out of habit. She has been thrown off the scent by someone with a flair for dissimulation.[4] But ethics often needs to be written as if everything is frozen in time in the case study or example. (There are deep problems here about the relationship between discursive practices and institutions, which Derrida has discussed in 'The Conflict of Faculties' (Derrida 1992).) Nevertheless, it needs to be recognised that in the practice of ethics things happen, circumstances change, and stories take new and unexpected twists.

So that is how it will be here: writing gives rise to more writing (Rorty 1978: 145). Others will point out all the shortcomings in what I say. Only if yet more writing results will I have been successful. Thus there will not be closure for the 'end' will find me pointing in more than one direction.[5] In the practice of ethics there is uncertainty: uncertainty about, among other things, the situation, what might happen and whether or not I did the right thing. Regrets, I've had a few, but then again, ethics seems to be written on the basis of *je ne regrette rien.*

There are features of this description of the way I am proceeding which I think some might describe as 'post.' I am trying to unpick the taken-for-granted idea – which goes unquestioned in the thinking of legislators – that information about a person necessarily is *their possession* and so is 'private'. I shall attempt to do this by showing that the confidential depends upon the possibility of revelation for its existence. However, it should perhaps be explained that if it turns out that this is a postal way of doing things, I would nevertheless not accept the ascription of 'post' in a periodising sense: I am not writing as if I assume that we live in a new kind of ethical period, a period following – as is sometimes said – a *coupure* of 1968. Rather it is that in some ways my approach is a moment or event that shares a characteristic modality with writing that is often, for want of better word,[6] called 'post' *whenever* it may occur. In this small way at least, I follow Jean-François Lyotard here: what is 'post' can come at any time, possibly before modernism, before structuralism. It can be its precursor. It is analysis, not as the breaking down into smaller parts but as a delving into (Lyotard 1993).[7] We proceed not by trying to show how the case fits into an ethical theory ('a legitimating grand narrative') but by offering analysis. Or, reverting to my already over-extended metaphor, let us try to set up some marker posts through the swamps.

Rough emotions

Considering, then, the place where I am, the subjective: first there was the state of mind aroused by the invitation to write this chapter and then there is the text that Anneke Lucassen has given us. I find myself beset by an unwelcome, almost overwhelming, crude utilitarianism. That utilitarianism is coloured by sympathy (not empathy[8]). This is sympathy, obviously, for Jane. Also, I feel for the general practitioners – of whom it is demanded that they be medical Enlightenment women and men – who have to face up to the responsibility and outcomes of action here in a way that I do not.

Let me try to explain what I mean by the instant, irresistible leap to utilitarianism. Surely, one says, Jane's predicament is so serious, and the possibility of needless suffering and disfigurement evident, that any calculation of the sum of human happiness must allow that Jane's predicament utterly outweighs the small gain for Phyllis that would derive from observing the proprieties of keeping Phyllis's test results secret. If Jane is privy to her test results, she can take a rational decision. Even if the result is that she has the same 'gene fault'[9] as Phyllis and she decides in prudence to undergo a mastectomy, she will do so with a much better understanding of the risks and without the debilitating worry that it might have been all entirely unnecessary. If she then goes ahead, her family will also be happier than they would have been had she had the mastectomy in ignorance of the full family history, as she is inclined to do simply to stop 'this gnawing anxiety constantly in the back of [my] head.' And so, at the beginning, I find myself saying, 'There's nothing to discuss, just *get on with it* and use Phyllis's genetic-test results.'

However, lots of things give me pause. Consider: this strangely powerful utilitarian response that presents itself as common sense, as *caused* by the situation and the humanity of the other within it, has all the force of a desire. Though for me, since I know none of the parties, the case should seem remote and abstract and separate from my doings, I nevertheless want to get in there and sort it out rationally. Let me cut through all this faffing about and inject a bit of management. Let me be in charge of bioethics – though come to think of it, giving me charge of all ethics and aesthetics would be best – and then we would soon see some action, some Top-Down Male Management (*my capitals*). Therefore beware: this is the will to power.

Let me say straight away that the force of this kind of utilitarian feeling ought not to be taken as evidence that utilitarianism gives the account of moral judgement. (Rather I am pointing out some seductions of utilitarianism.) All the problems associated with trying to pin down what constitutes happiness, the role and nature of pleasure in moral thought, whether it might not be better to be bovine and satisfied than reflective and dissatisfied, why some people will end productive living in a search to secure the short-term pleasure that drugs will bring, are all well-worn disputes that rattle on. There is little meeting ground between the engaging intellectual dissatisfactions of the Oxford quad and the pressing concerns of higher education in the developing world, much less the brute struggle for survival of much of the world's population (Withers 1997). The conclusion that happiness is culture bound, relative to place and time, is hard to deny.

The effect of all these millennia of discussion, a properly postal state of affairs, is that every apparently simple example that might make me spring to a utilitarian position will be subject to further discussion and disagreement. Even for the committed utilitarian there is no escape from continuing and continual examination of each and every new case. Utilitarianism does not produce ready answers. Casey's (1971) discussion of an obstetrician faced with a choice of letting a woman giving birth die and the child live, or vice versa, shows that even the most apparently straightforward case can give rise to prolonged debate about the features of action, and how ethics might proceed, without agreement ever being reached.

Refinement

Initially I thought that the GPs were taking that same crude utilitarian stance. They seemed to be saying 'It's clear what should be done and Phyllis won't even know that we've used her tests.' But when I read the case again, more carefully, it appears that they did not jump immediately to this simple solution. No, they have taken into account British General Medical Council (GMC) guidelines that (in the text, as reported by the GPs) say 'we should only break confidentiality in a serious or life-threatening condition.' Well, is this perhaps just a less crude, more refined form, rule-utilitarianism? They seem to enjoin following the rule, that is the GMC rule, other things being equal (*ceteris paribus*). The idea is that greater good can be assured in the long term if confidentiality is maintained. This will be an especially greater good since it will be known that, all other things being equal, this rule is everywhere observed. Only if this is a case of a serious or life-threatening condition will other things not be equal.

The advantage of rule-utilitarianism is that it seems to give us a get-out from crudity in that it allows us in certain cases to override the first results of the utilitarian calculus. But the *difficulty* with it is that in any particular case where we try to show that following the rule will everywhere outweigh the other kinds of happiness involved, we find that there are no objective ways of doing so. We decide how to act on other unstated or subjective grounds. That this is not just an empirical finding but a feature of practical reasoning has been argued by philosophers many times, and well. It is just about impossible to determine in what circumstances it can be calculated whether implementing the rule, coupled with knowledge that the rule has been followed, outweighs or fails to outweigh the consequences of ignoring the rule. And looking at Jane's case we can see that we have no idea how or why confidentiality would outweigh the possibility of Jane's pain and disfigurement, or her potential happiness if it is discovered that she does not have the gene fault. What I want to ask is, *why* should it be more important that people in general should know that their data will be hidden away uselessly than that Jane should be spared possibly needless disfigurement? (The refined would no doubt reply 'Isn't it more important that people in general know that their confidentiality will be respected?')

Notoriously, the *ceteris paribus* clause is problematic for rule-utilitarianism. Here we have it sourced from the GMC in a deeply puzzling form: 'except in the case of serious or life-threatening conditions.' Seriousness is negotiable but can we be sure whether or not this is a case involving life and death? Opinions seem to be divided between Jane, who seems quite certain that she has learned that it is, and some medics who say it is not. The geneticist, for example, says that though the risk of cancer is significantly reduced there are not yet data on mortality following this kind of operation. In rule-utilitarian terms, what the rule seems to mean is that confidentiality is hedonistic, yet consequences, such as the threat to life, must nevertheless somehow be attended to. By this point, the many questions concerning how these different considerations can all be weighed and how the problems of action can be resolved have become as difficult to disentangle as a knot in the fur of a Persian cat.

It is sometimes said that postmodern morality is aestheticised ethics of taste (Rorty 1986, Shusterman 1988). It seems to me that *any* ethical position that neglected serious consequences of action, such as the causing of pain or threat to life, would be aesthetic or evasive or in some sense unconcerned with the basic core of morality. In saying this I have in mind the curious remark of the geneticist who proposes that it should be made a condition of having the test that agreement is given by the subject that the results can be shared with family members. This, we are told, would be likely to prevent 'people like Phyllis taking the test in the first place, so Jane would be no better off, *but at least we wouldn't be in the difficult dilemma we are in now*' (my italics). Coupled with the claim quoted from the GPs: 'It wouldn't have been an issue, of course, had the two women not been registered at our practice',[10] these remarks seem to me to place value on escape from dilemmas over consequences, yet have been proposed by people who have shown sensitivity to ethical issues.

Here there is an inviting path that we shall surely be tempted to take. As resisting readers we will desire to find escape from the dilemma in the case study. We will, without acknowledging the fact, look for reasons for claiming that Jane's situation is really not what it seems or what she makes it out to be. We shall insist that Phyllis can be brought to change her mind and allow her test results to be revealed. But hang on, isn't a willingness to confront dilemmas and a concern for consequences often said to be central to moral reasoning? It will be important to recognise the action of this resistance in our reading and to assess how far these comforting thoughts are well founded or whether the probability is that the consequences will, after all, be just as Jane would describe them.

If a concern for this kind of consequence might be said to lie at the centre of moral deliberation, it does not follow that the surrounding ethical territory, and especially what is to be found at the margins,[11] is necessarily consequentialist. Consequentialism is in any case beset by the same issues that were discussed above, arising out of the nature of human agency and responsibility. It is the nature of practical reasoning that when we decide, we cannot have a 'full' description of circumstances, cannot be certain of the consequences and there will be unintended consequences. Nevertheless, either something is done or it is not done.[12] The idea of ethical deliberation is that it is about agency.

I introduced this discussion not to denounce the utilitarian approach but to recognise its strong hold on our thinking and to realise that, nevertheless, it cannot be the whole of thinking. (It cannot dominate, as the postal workers say.) Furthermore, I want to begin to uncover the importance of ideas about confidentiality and data in all this. How confidentiality is construed, as being necessary to the good life, or as some kind of good in itself, or as the proper thing to do – a kind of aesthetic for living – is at the moment mysterious. The production of these delicacies needs analysis.

Similarly, I shall not tarry while investigating human rights, duties, descriptivism, or other such approaches since they did not seize my thinking in the same way. Just note that 'rights' do not seem to get a better grip on the case. It is always difficult to see what the source of 'rights' is supposed to be. Reviewing the changing history of rights, they appear to be a convenient philosophical label, or legal shorthand summary, of where innumerable power struggles have reached so far. Thus there seems to be no evident logic in the relationship of rights one to another. Recently we have seen 'the right to refuse treatment' has been upheld but the apparently closely related 'right to end one's life' or the 'right to arrange the bringing about of a dignified death' has been denied. In our case, Jane's 'right to have the best information and treatment about her disease' conflicts with Phyllis's 'right to confidentiality'. As we shall see, confidentiality about genes is strange enough when construed as a right, but the notion of a right that admits of exceptions, such as 'in a very serious or life-threatening condition', is fraught with difficulty.

Practically reasoning

Reading the text seems to propel us towards a particular account of Jane as someone who, after listening, reading, discussing and reflecting, has decided on a course of action. She relates her meeting with a woman who has had a prophylactic mastectomy and so sees this operation as practical, something that could be arranged and soon. However, that does not of itself mean that she has made a firm decision: characteristically people will get to this stage of having taken a decision but have doubts, change their minds, change them back again and discuss with significant others who bring in a different perspective and other considerations.

It could be the case that Jane is using the possibility of a mastectomy as a negotiating tool. The meeting between Phyllis and Jane is necessarily empty of detail. It seems likely that Jane went to see her aunt expecting to find out Phyllis's condition. Both players could have some thoughts that remain unacknowledged. One assumes that they will each have had a script, prepared in imagination by playing out scenarios, which will then have been lost as soon as the meeting took place: unfortunately, everyone's script is always different.[13] We cannot know but the point is that we cannot be sure that a 'major and mutilating piece of surgery' will be a consequence of retained confidentiality about Phyllis's test results. But these problems about the uncertain nature of the human condition, consequences and agency cannot be solved by adopting a methodology of enriching the textual detail without end. To be practical, let's just agree or accept that the discussions between Jane and Phyllis and their advisers could be interminable – understandings deepening, clarifying or just clouding – were it not for the nature of time.

It has been my experience that time is not an unlimited resource in the life of surgeons, GPs or even counsellors, yet time and the experience of time is absent from case studies which must be frozen at a certain point. Disturbances to situations, decisions and actions all have this nasty habit of taking place in time and under experienced time pressures. If there is a surgeon who will agree to operate and Jane consents then an operation could be arranged. It might go ahead and then something irrevocable at a given time will have happened. If it were not for the fact that cancers either appear or do not appear in time then discussion could go on endlessly but if the operation could forestall cancer then it would need to be finished before cancer appeared. If one of the parties tells Jane the results of Phyllis's results, then again, something irreversible will actually have happened; someone will have acted and discussion will move on, to be about what was done and what should happen next. Some practical reasoning will have been effected. This will be different from a good deal of something that resembles it: practically practical reasoning. It is, of course, important to clarify stories, enrich understandings and to discuss details and accounts. It can be enjoyable philosophically, therapeutically, imaginatively and so on, but in practice someone or some thing, or even the discussion itself, will have changed the world.

People act in changing circumstances, their actions change the circumstances. I am not just signalling a concern for 'what is to be done'. The dilemma of ethical reflection is this: the constative takes time, time to be discursive, to bear repetition and to establish an element of generalisability without the pressures of the performative; but if the force of time and the effects of agency are absent, ethical discussion becomes ahistorical.

Rationalism

Is the seductive power of utilitarianism that, in contrast to other philosophical positions, it seems to force itself upon us as a practical and *rational* calculus for decision-making, allowing us to come to a decision in time?

Those writers who assume a periodising sense of 'post' frequently cite the end of the Enlightenment idea of human progress by the shorthand term 'Auschwitz' (see Lyotard's discussion in Lyotard 1993). After the Holocaust, who can advocate rationalism? The difficulty is that we conflate rationality with having a *good* reason, and having a good reason we equate with being wholly justified. Through so much of the last century we saw that reason can be used to pursue just about any ends and ingenious reasoning can be used to justify it. The Fascist governments were modernisers who used technological reasoning to pursue their wholly evil ends. Kenneth Branagh, explaining his role in a BBC television drama as Heydrich at the Wannsee Conference of 20 January 1942, constructed from Eichmann's notes, said 'My reaction was jaw-dropping astonishment at the tone of this meeting and the apparently easy, casual quality to the discussion of the fate of an entire race across Europe. It felt like the quiet political in-fighting of a board meeting at a big company' (*Radio Times*, 2002).

Those who use 'post' in a periodising sense urge that we have *now* seen the end of grand narratives, the end of history. Yet grand rationalising narratives are still around. 'The emerging world-wide *imposition* of democracy and democratic ways of life' is itself a grand narrative. The presumption is that to impose a particular kind of democracy, whether by economic or military force, is a rational thing to do. But the paradox of this imposition and form of decision-making is that these same democratic governments have used force to support dictators of many kinds wherever it suited them and have assisted in replacing a democratically elected government with a military dictatorship. 'Those who are not with us are against us' (recently glossed as 'whoever is not with us – on the side of good – is against us – opting for evil') is a profoundly undemocratic remark yet springs readily to the speech of those who would impose their particular form of democracy. But let me quickly explain that I am *not* commenting on this to make any political points of any kind: I simply wish, in as quick a way as possible, to remind us of the seductive power of rationalism and the instant appeal of a rational decision-making calculus, which I am suggesting is illusory.

Nevertheless, to be 'post' is not to be relativist in the sense of holding that everything is local and anything goes. Certainly there is evil in the world. I am pointing to the process that allows the exercise and maintenance of power to go disguised as justifiable, rational policing. This is politics as the concealing of the means to power under a cloak called rationality, a process sometimes itself concealed by use of the innocuous-sounding term 'spin'.

I used to think that John Rawls's veil of ignorance wrapped everything up ethically in rationality (Rawls 1972: especially 136–7). We ask, what would we choose not knowing who we were to be and what our position in the world would be? Rationality would dictate prudence. Unfortunately, the practicalities of this are manifold. I shall point to just two of them of concern here: first, if we are periodising 'post' then we live in a time when people opt for the lottery in all aspects of life in preference to any kind of redistribution; second, under the veil Jane would decide that in Phyllis's place she would reveal the information but Phyllis – whether or not she is under the veil – comes to the opposite conclusion. What we want to do in our interest, or in order to pursue power, can be endlessly and selfishly justified on rational, universalising grounds.[14]

A gymnasium called sculptors

You will see that my method is to try you by exhausting the other possibilities.

Since I first read Ryle I have been impressed by the idea of a category mistake (Ryle 1949). It sounds good; it sounds easy. Has Phyllis made a category mistake about her body? Has the GMC made a mistake about bodies in general in advising confidentiality?

Phyllis seems to think of her body, or anything to do with her body, as her possession. It is to be guarded and kept from others if she chooses. It can be used in family wars. Recently in Britain we have seen how even the parts of dead children are regarded as the property of their parents. All this is so widely assumed to be self-evidently right that my suggestion that there could be some kind of mistake will seem wild. Therefore, let me make the case out from a less familiar quarter.

We talk about a duty to oneself to keep one's body in good shape, to stay fit and healthy. Some treatments have been refused to smokers who do not acknowledge this duty, or at least do not fulfil it. But then, on television, I have seen competitions where body-builders exhibit their torsos and assume poses to show off certain groups of muscles. Many people express repulsion at seeing men and women showing off stringy sets of enlarged muscles but the body-builders talk of their bodies as sculptural objects, which they work on. In order to achieve particular results, some of them are willing to take steroids, even at the risk of damaging those same bodies. The postmodernist Arnold Schwarzenegger, model of pure hard android near-machine, was reported as having taken steroids leading to heart problems. So the body-builders have rejected the ideal of fitness and health for the idealism of an aesthetic object to be worked on, even if it will not then last as long as it might without the work. And so, in Portsmouth on my way to the ferry I saw a gymnasium called 'Sculptors'.

Isn't there some kind of mistake here? Aren't they thinking about their bodies under the wrong category? While you are alive, your body is not some sort of possession to be worked on or used by someone else as an object: it is *you*. After your death, it could be different.

One can see the attraction of this kind of argument for sorting out issues about the appropriate conceptualisations of persons, including, of course, Ryle's corrective to a certain Cartesianism of 'the ghost in the machine'. This is suggestive of possibilities for medical ethics in considerations to do with persons and their bodies, as in the case of Phyllis and Jane. In a sense, if Phyllis's living body is Phyllis then it is a mistake to think that it can be hidden as a private possession; she reveals herself in all that she does. Certain characteristics and conditions are on display, so what choice could there be, appropriately, over what is hidden, guarded and secreted?

This seems to me to be an important thought. Though I shall return to investigate this issue below, unfortunately the category mistake is much too slender as a language tool to do much heavy-duty work. (Sorry, I slipped into Ryle-speak.) There could be examples from medicine, maybe surgery, where, far from constituting a category mistake, it would be appropriate and perhaps important at some point to conceptualise the person as an object, a body. (I do not recall reading any account of how the surgeon views the subject when he or she operates but I am assuming here that some detachment from the thought that the body is a person must be necessary.) My own counter-example, however, occurs to me more directly from considerations of sculp-ture: the traditional artist's model *is* an object; he, she or more properly, it, must be an object, immobile, not interacting, observed.

The very possibility of choosing to reveal things about ourselves depends upon the possibility of hiding other things. It's not much help to say that it is a conceptual mistake to hide a part of the body as if it were an inanimate object. I have no intention of arguing that anyone who is not a naturist is making a category mistake. Nevertheless, though this path was a dead-end, I am left with a disorienting feeling that somewhere around here some interesting connections may lie.

Trust me, I'm your psychiatrist

Unless we make strenuous efforts to escape it, the case study presents a dilemma. We might say that it is Jane's dilemma but it has the form of two general propositions about confidentiality, both of which seem to be correct:
1. confidentiality is essential;
2. confidentiality should be denied.

In the study, a number of players try to give priority to confidentiality while stitching the tear between 1 and 2 in different ways. One way is to invoke the GMC proposed exceptions to confidentiality. This might be urged as a kind of rule-utilitarianism but, importantly, medics increasingly criticised or operating in a litigious environment might adopt it out of prudence. Another approach is to insist that trust *means* guarding confidentiality and that trust is more important than the trauma of mastectomy. I attempt a different resolution by maintaining, contrary to what is taken for granted, that trust is not bound up in maintaining confidentiality. Thus I would not allow that proposition 1 – Confidentiality is essential – is to be accorded dominance as a principle over 2 – Confidentiality should be denied. To maintain this I need to examine the nature of confidentiality and to show how data seemed to become the possession of the patient but also I should point out that 'trust' is not a simple matter.

It is often said that the idea of the professional as an expert has led to much abuse. We have trusted the physician, the teacher and the solicitor to act wholly and solely in our interests as an individual in their care. That this trust has sometimes been misplaced and that the dependency of the trusting subject has been used a base for the power of the professional is undeniable, but this is a complicated set of relationships. The simple fix of recasting the relationship as consumer and supplier, with the consumer as the authority on her own best interests, is crude and conceals many important distinctions.

I need to trust the physician to endeavour to cure me and, where it is possible, to restore me to health, to do all that he or she can to restore me. The physician should administer drugs appropriately, not give me a lethal dose of morphine when an aspirin is all that is required to put me right or when

I have simply come for a check-up and I am in reasonable condition. I need to trust the physician to continue to study and learn and to take pains to find the correct diagnosis in difficult circumstances. These are the things that a physician must do. If the physician breaks this kind of trust, then I should fail to trust him or her in all things. If the physician breaks confidentiality, however, it does *not* follow that I should not then trust him or her to do the things that a physician must do.

The difficulty and range of these cases and the role in it of the patient is a highly complicated matter. The part played by physicians in eugenics stands as a warning against oversimplification. Just by way of illustration of the complexity, consider the case reported some years ago of a patient receiving treatment for a psychiatric condition who shattered the glass of a fish and chip shop and hurled abuse at the owner. The police were called. The 'patient' was shouting to the neighbourhood that his wife and the owner of the shop were having an affair. His psychiatrist treated him on the basis that this was another delusion but, of course, it transpired that it was not.

I should be able to trust my physician in certain circumstances to break confidentiality about my anxiety and depression to make sure that my family understands what is happening to me, does not simply reject me and is able to ensure that I take the tablets. I need to trust the physician to do the right thing despite my insistence that he or she should do the wrong thing. Though safeguards are built on the assumption that I am the ultimate authority on right and wrong simply because things are happening to me, this is not necessarily always the case.

The model of consumer is now so pervasive that we incline to read criticism into the actions of the oncologist in sending off the BRCA genetic test on Phyllis. He seems defensive. But, as he explains, the patient consents to lots of investigative tests. I should trust that, if I need an operation, my surgeon will arrange a battery of tests and not ask me to approve each and every test. The requirement to reveal hitherto secret details about the way in which post-mortems are carried out on infant corpses has led to a reluctance to perform them. Medics are becoming increasingly cautious and so will become ever less ready to consider the range of possibilities presented. Something important and good can be lost to caution.

Proprieties

Where are the results of the test? Are they marks on paper in drawers in filing cabinets or instructions in some coding for a computer? More or less material, probably they are not physically in Phyllis's possession, yet they appear to be hers. She can say who can see them, except that she cannot say which doctors can or may not see them. Is the National Health Service (NHS) in Britain a kind of bank? It guards her document in a secure vault but necessarily allows its employees to look at them.

These valuable documents were not given by Phyllis to the NHS to hold for her; I doubt that she has held them in her hands. More probably, someone capable of making a selection (editing) told her what was there. She did not, she says, even ask for them to be created. So why are they hers? Not, it seems, by virtue of authorship, signature, purchase or arrangement.[15]

As you would expect, I have thought about privacy in the sense of keeping others out by means of high walls and broken glass, guards and title deeds; covering the signpost over and having the power to prevent others from uncovering it; pointing all the signposts in the wrong directions to fool the invading forces, which presupposes that one knows the right directions. (This leads to reflections on the supposed materiality of the signifier – well at least the signpost is material – problems of ostension and what those place names on the signpost signify.) I have in contemplation compared those who turn signposts round with geographers – who have a compulsion to map the right way to everywhere – educators and others whose mission is to reveal rather than to hide. I have thought about the primacy of writing or speech with respect to privacy and confidentiality, that little matter of deniability, evidence, opportunity and corroboration. Now that the ink-jet printer has replaced the individuality of each typewriter face, deniability is increased and obfuscation improves the prospects of defending confidentiality. But none of this is sufficiently similar to the case in hand to throw light in any direction. I am forced back to that constant irritation, the feeling that establishing how control over the information is obtained and guarded must be the clue to *why* it is maintained, and hence what I think about it.

Authorship of information is the normal way into its control. In the extreme case, that privilege of privacy within one's head suggests opportunities for control. Of course we know that the private thoughts in the head can be revealed by mistake, through blurting out,[16] through one's facial expression, or a chain of deduction or association. Still, choice over to what to reveal is the norm. Hence the possibilities for confiding in someone depend upon the possibility of privacy. But we know from the private-language argument that the possibility of private thought depends upon the public. The oddity in the present case is that we are told that issues of confidentiality arise, yet there is no sense in which Phyllis chooses to confide in someone else or not: she does not produce the information for herself and then choose whether or not to confide in someone, rather she is told of its existence without asking for it. Similarly, we might be told of the existence of information about us, concerning, say, credit ratings.

If we think of the test results as information, then the right to a say in its distribution appears to flow from the consideration that Phyllis is denoted by the signifiers and something is predicated of her. But does that give everyone who is denoted in information rights over that information? It is difficult to come up with a reason why it should, though it seems that there ought to be some connection with an opportunity at least to comment upon information that could do us harm. I seem here to be moving in line with ideas about justice. However, the idea of confidentiality invoked in this case does not seem to have been solely with respect to matters that might harm Phyllis but rather for all and every information about her medical condition, unless a serious or life-threatening condition should be involved. Thus we are driven back to those strange ideas about the body and how to think about it in terms of privacy, belonging and confidentiality, but this time with respect to 'information'.

How close can one come to thinking of the body as a text or corpus?[17] Isn't DNA information and hence a text to be read? Well we certainly talk about reading a person's facial expression. We can look at someone and think that they probably have a particular condition and be fairly sure that they have a particular disease. Imagine that I have a bodily condition I find distressing: call it baldness. Anyone looking at me can read it but I would like to keep it confidential. I wish to hide it under a toupee. Now I have to confide in the wigmaker. So, like the bankers, this is a class of person who must be trusted to guard confidences. I have to have confidence in him. There remain so many ways for my 'secret' – that piece of information I wish to conceal, to secrete away – yet to be revealed. A high wind, a swimming pool, a close reader who detects the join, someone who works for the wigmaker and likes to gossip, can all render my confidence misplaced. It is part of the nature of confidence that it can be shattered, of trust that it can be broken, of confidentiality that it is subject to discovery and revelation. Why, then, should I attempt to guard it? Shouldn't we argue for all to be revealed?

Some genetic information might be used against us. Insurance companies would dearly love to obtain the kind of genetic information that Jane seeks. If they had access to that kind of information, they would be better placed to refuse life or health insurance to certain classes of people and so would increase profits for their shareholders and hence maximise human happiness. So here we have an example where genetic information should be confidential. Just as I do not want my bank to profit from the use of information of my account by selling to their 'partners' overseas, where data-protection rules may not be as strongly protective as in Britain, neither would I want an insurance company to profit from reading my genes. But I do not want to set up another totalising rule, such that 'information should be freely available, except in cases where a third party would profit materially', since this approach would fall foul of the same kind of issues I discussed earlier. All the different kinds of cases need careful excavation.

We are familiar with incidents where information that a politician or celebrity regards as confidential, such as sexual preferences, has been exposed to the media with the danger of some kind of harm resulting to their career. Some politicians and other celebrities have found themselves 'outed' over having cancer. Just the very fact of having cancer seems to be, for some people, a secret to be guarded. Breast cancer could be a particularly sensitive piece of information for women because that part of the female anatomy can have a key role in the social construction of femininity. Similarly, a man suffering from breast cancer might wish to conceal the fact because masculinity is opposed to the idea that not only women develop breast cancer. These ideas about self could, then, cause an insistence on confidentiality of information. It becomes *sensitised*, no longer just neutral.

We think naturally of these cases. Thus a spokesperson for the Human Genetics Commission urged that it should be an offence to obtain and analyse DNA samples without permission. This is to think of the samples solely as a part of the body that is taken away. Thus any permission has to be given by the rest of the body, but it was also said that this recommendation was intended to protect privacy. The sound-bite could not, of course, be an accurate summary. When trying to evade paternity claims, it would be useful to insist on privacy. Rapists have evaded detection for long periods by substituting a sample, provided by an obliging friend, for their own. Here the sample is pertinent information, not just a part of the body. We surely cannot uphold the privacy of rapists withholding this information and cannot straightforwardly support privacy and confidentiality in every case.

As has been pointed out elsewhere in this book, the text is not explicit whether it is known in the family that Phyllis has experienced breast cancer, but there are strong indications that this is known. Perhaps it could be read from Phyllis. In any case, the high incidence of breast cancer in the family would militate against there being any reason why Phyllis should want to hide from Jane the fact of her breast cancer, if it were not already known. In all that Phyllis says there is no indication that she would see that knowledge as an issue. Nor does it appear that she sees the results of her test as confidential due to being sensitive and related to her feminine identity. The reasons she gives are quite different.

The sleep of unreason

Here is something rather extraordinary: 'It was my result, not anyone else's business.' To say something is none of your business is to say it is something you should not be active about. The test result is a vital matter for Jane, so why should she not be active about it? How can Phyllis decide this for Jane? It is to say 'This is not something that you can engage in through useful or profitable exchange; you have nothing to give me in exchange for this.' Phyllis is thinking, therefore, of services rendered by Phyllis in the past for which nothing was given in exchange. She was not, she now in effect says, offering her care for the dying as love, as a gift without strings. She expected to be recompensed, put into the will. The business arrangement, which Phyllis implies should have been there but was not effected, was not confined to the individuals who were cared for but was also with other family members, though they were not aware of its existence.

The issue is not whether or not it is known that Phyllis has had breast cancer. (And if this were not known, it could probably be read by Jane from the family circumstances and Phyllis's place in it.) The question to be settled is whether or not the test results can be revealed to Jane. Imagine the following scenarios in different circumstances, in other possible worlds:

1. Jane knows that Phyllis has the gene fault and the form it takes;
2. Jane knows that Phyllis does not have the gene fault;
3. Jane does not know whether Phyllis has the gene fault, or the form it takes if she has it.

In worlds 1 and 2, in many ways Phyllis is untouched that Jane has the knowledge that she has, but Jane is empowered. So it is that empowerment that affects Phyllis: she sees Jane empowered. In world 3 Phyllis has the power. It is this world which Phyllis wishes to maintain. Concealing the results from Jane, 'respecting confidentiality', would then be assisting Phyllis to maintain her power to damage Jane, not some other thing. If a legislator says something like 'If counselling does not persuade someone to consent to sharing information with their relatives the individual's decision to withhold information should be paramount,' then the legislator is doing violence to someone like Jane.

Should counselling be persuasion? A common assumption here is that if people can just get together and the thing can be talked through, then subjects like Phyllis are likely to be persuaded. If they are not, then there must be a good, rational explanation for their wish to maintain confidentiality and so their wishes should be respected. I see no signs that Phyllis will have a sensible talk about everything. Consider what she says: 'They were interested in my relations, which was *a bit of cheek*'; 'I don't feel I *owe them* anything'; 'It was my result, not anyone else's *business*'; 'I'm fed up with *being blamed* for anything that goes wrong in our family.' I would say that this is the *business* of resistance. It is not, of course, uncommon for people to feel guilty when a loved one or someone who they have been caring for dies, even though they are in no way responsible for the death. Guilt can be a factor even when there has been no physical connection at the time of death, as when someone says of a brother killed in a distant car crash, 'I felt as if I had dropped him.' Derrida points out the important role of guilt in resistance (Derrida 1998) and guilt can be described by the subject as 'I'm fed up with being blamed.'

The point that I wish to draw attention to, through all this talk about resistance, is that the dislocation of madness from unreason, or at least a breaking of the unity of that connection, which Foucault demonstrates, has pushed towards an assumption that all kinds of unconscious or unacknowledged thought processes can be made available to consciousness through relatively straightforward rational means. I am not suggesting in any way whatsoever that Phyllis is mad:[18] I am trying to draw attention in a forceful way to how far we have slipped in analysis towards writing as if all relevant material can be uncovered through reasonable discussion or counselling so that we need only present our analysis to the subjects and it will be patiently accepted.

Perhaps I ought not to have slipped in (subliminally?) the idea of Phyllis as a patient. Nevertheless, since we cannot be complicit with her exercise of power that causes harm to Jane and with her violence to Jane (and so will not regard the information as Phyllis's own, giving sole *owner*ship, but will reveal the results to Jane), counselling needs to be conceptualised differently from persuasion of a reasonable person well motivated to do good. It should not take the form of a vain attempt to persuade Phyllis to agree to cooperate. Nothing should be expected of Phyllis in return. The offer of counselling should be made as a gift: a true gift would not require reciprocation but would be given freely. We cannot guarantee the right outcome for Phyllis but we are not responsible for her refusal to accept our analysis (Derrida 1998). Phyllis will find it difficult to accept that her care of her dying relatives can be an act of love and that no blame attaches to us for our inherited genetic make-up. She will see it as unfair that she was not thanked in a will. But where does it say it has to be fair (Heller 1984)?

NOTES

1 I steal this expression of resistance from Jacques Derrida (1998: 25) to signal that I make substantial borrowings from that volume, and perhaps also in the hope of emulating Derrida's gracious way of evading the logic of the constraints placed upon him by the organisers of symposia.

2 Spivak (Derrida 1976, English translation) has 'We must begin wherever we are and the thought of the trace, which cannot not take the scent [the original French is *flair*] into account, has already taught us that it was impossible to justify a point of departure absolutely. Wherever we are: in a text where we already believe ourselves to be.' It will be noted that in the text I have strayed very slightly from this standard translation.

3 I am neither originally French nor do I disagree with anyone. And if you disagree with that . . .

4 Rorty (1978) says 'The most shocking thing about Derrida's work is his use of multilingual puns, joke etymologies, allusions from anywhere, and phonic and typographical gimmicks' (Rorty 1978: 146–7). Since in this chapter I am attempting to offer a Socratic *pharmakon*, and in a discussion of ethics should acknowledge my sources, and since Derrida extensively explains the importance of this kind of

writing, I must therefore blame Derrida for my shocking French/English puns (see '*flair*' above), dubious etymologies and allusions.

5 I have illustrated desiderata about beginnings, introductions, conclusions, endings and 'typographical gimmicks' in Withers (1997).

6 There is little doubt that the expressions 'postmodernism' and 'post-structuralism' have proved highly misleading for many readers because they necessarily seem to mean something temporal or periodising. Perhaps the idea of a new period has added glamour and led to media exposure such that it is now too late to change the expressions in order to avoid further confusion. Use of the terms has also encouraged helpful puns and theorising about post-Post Office and postal services.

7 Derrida (1998, Chapter 1 'Resistances') has a more detailed and extended explanation of analysis in much the same sense as it used by Lyotard.

8 Sympathy is widely misunderstood: it is a wholly good thing, unlike empathy, which doesn't exist. Probably.

9 Throughout I shall use this loaded expression 'gene fault' as shorthand for the complicated geneology explained so well by Anneke Lucassen.

10 They say 'of course' but their reasoning here is not clear to me: if they mean simply that they would have been in ignorance of the existence of Phyllis's test had she been in another practice, then the genetic record would have been kept unhelpfully pigeon-holed in a way that raises other important issues. Throughout this whole case study there is a theme of practitioners wishing to serve the interests of a single patient, to act as the barrister for Phyllis only or for Jane only.

11 In ethical debate, people often become unnecessarily agitated by the use of the metaphors 'core' and 'at the margin'. As Derrida frequently points out, one cannot talk of being at the centre without an awareness of the margins and at the margins is often where the interest lies. Anyone whose neighbour will not restrict the height of evergreens and sycamore knows the importance of boundary disputes.

12 This is not intended as a tautology. By 'not done' here I have in mind avoided, neglected, forgotten, resisted, left too late, botched, put to one side and so on.

13 You will ask, how do I know this? Would it work if I said that I deduced it from personal observation?

14 Mike Parker remarked to me recently that Rawls depends upon a Piagetian developmental structuralism. This might suggest that for Rawls people who, instead of operating under the veil, conceal their own interests under a cloak of rationality are not operating at the fully developed stage.

15 Mysteriously, the geneticist says 'I feel that in these situations, Phyllis's test result really belongs to her whole family, not just to her.' What constitutes her 'whole family' and how these results belong them would be interesting to explore.

16 In court, I was surprised to hear that a man accused of murdering his wife in their bedroom had shortly afterwards that night visited the pub and in a loud voice told his friends all about how he strangled her with the cords of a lamp. He pleaded 'Not guilty' to murder due to mistaken identity in the dark, the lamp being inoperative, due to the wires having been pulled out of their clamps. Though this is the extreme example, chatting about matters which one intended to keep secret is not uncommon.

17 These puns draw together some important threads: the very etymology of text as tissue demonstrates just how closely this is all woven together.

18 Though I do know of families where, confronted with a case of a family member who refuses to be reasonable and attributes apparently random accusations of blame and so on, someone would say 'She's mad, she is.'

REFERENCES

Barthes, R. (1973). *Mythologies.* London: Paladin.

Casey, J. (1971). Actions and consequences. In J. Casey, *Morality and Moral Reasoning.* London: Methuen, 155–205.

Derrida, J. (1967). *De la grammatologie.* Paris: Minuit. (English translation: Spivak, G. C. (1976). *Of Grammatology.* Baltimore: Johns Hopkins University Press).

(1992). Mochlos or the conflict of the faculties. In R. Rand, ed., *Logomachia: The Conflict of the Faculties.* Lincoln, Nebr. and London: University of Nebraska Press, 1–34.

(1998). *Resistances of Psychoanalysis.* (English translation: Kamuf, P., Brault, P.-A. and Nass, M. Stanford, Calif.: California University Press.) [Originally published in French 1996.]

Heller, J. (1984). *God Knows.* London: Cape.

Lyotard, J.-F. (1993). Note on the meaning of 'post-'. In T. Docherty, ed., *Postmodernism: A Reader.* Hemel Hempstead: Harvester, 47–50.

Radio Times. (2002). 19–25 January, 36.

Rawls, J. (1972). *A Theory of Justice.* Oxford: Oxford University Press.

Rorty, R. (1978). Philosophy as a kind of writing: an essay on Derrida. *N Lit Hist,* **10,** 141–60.

Rorty, R. (1986). Freud and moral reflection. In J. H. Smith and W. Kerrigan, eds., *Pragmatism's Freud: The Moral Disposition of Psychoanalysis.* Baltimore: Johns Hopkins University Press, 1–27.

Ryle, G. (1949). *The Concept of Mind.* London: Hutchinson.

Shusterman, R. (1988). Postmodernist aestheticism: a new moral philosophy? *Theory, Culture & Society,* **5,** 337–55.

Withers, R. (1997). If on a winter's night an editor . . . *Teaching Higher Ed,* **2**(3), 219–24.

8

A utilitarian approach

Julian Savulescu

What is utilitarianism?

Utilitarianism is, on one level, a straightforward moral theory (Savulescu 2003). According to utilitarians, all that matters is well-being. The more well-being, the better. The right action is that action that results in the greatest sum total of well-being.

Utilitarianism has several strengths. It does not invoke mysterious or vague concepts like rights, duties (e.g. to some deity), enlightenment (e.g. of the Truth), liberation (e.g. of the worker), which are difficult to define plausibly or apply consistently and appropriately in practice. It invokes the most basic of concepts: that our lives can become better or worse. Our lives become worse, for example, when we die prematurely of some illness. And people's actions are wrong when they make our lives become worse.

Utilitarianism protects the welfare of the individual. People should not be harmed in the name of some ideal or human construct. One needs a very good reason to harm people, according to utilitarianism. Those reasons would have to do with great benefits to other people.

Application

Lucassen writes that in clinical genetics 'there can be a direct conflict between preserving the confidentiality of one patient and the right of other family members to know information about their genetic status and risk of disease.'

It is notoriously difficult to define a right and balance different rights and interests. What is the 'right of a family member to know information about their genetic status'? Where do such rights come from? How are they to be balanced against the duty to protect confidentiality?

Utilitarians find all this rather mysterious. For them, the main issue is how the various courses of action (in this case, disclosing or not disclosing

Case Analysis in Clinical Ethics, ed. Richard Ashcroft, Anneke Lucassen, Michael Parker, Marian Verkerk, Guy Widdershoven. Published by Cambridge University Press.

confidential information against the wishes of a person) will affect the lives of the parties concerned. If Phyllis's information is disclosed to Jane, what will be the consequences for the well-being of Phyllis and Jane? And if the information is not disclosed, how will each person's life unfold?

Consider the impact on each of disclosure. The broad interests that Jane has in disclosure are those related to either:

1. avoiding breast cancer (by having a prophylactic mastectomy if she tests positive);
2. avoiding an unnecessary operation of prophylactic bilateral mastectomy (if she tests negative).

The harm to Phyllis of disclosure is the negative psychological consequences (distress, feelings of being blamed, unhappiness, depression, etc.) that would follow disclosure.

Regardless of the test result (i.e. whether it is positive or negative), Jane has a significant interest in having access to genetic testing. She either avoids breast cancer or an unnecessary mastectomy. Breast cancer is terrible in many ways: not only are there physical consequences that cause pain and death, but significant psychological and social consequences, with the disruption of normal life and the frustration of most plans that a woman has for her life. A bilateral mastectomy is also very bad. It is a major surgical procedure with a (small) risk of death related to anaesthesia and significant postoperative complications (bleeding, infection, pain, etc.) with long-term disfigurement and significant psychological and social consequences.

The harm to Phyllis is likely to be much less. She has little contact with her family as it is, so there is little to be lost in terms of positive existing family relationships. She may suffer some distress but this is likely to be much less than the harm that Jane would suffer from breast cancer or an unnecessary mastectomy.

Consider now the consequences of not disclosing the result. Jane is contemplating a prophylactic mastectomy in the absence of a confirmed positive gene test. Let us assume that she goes ahead with this. There is a fifty per cent chance that this procedure will be unnecessary. The benefit of not disclosing the result is that Phyllis achieves what she wants and her psychological equilibrium is maintained. But again, a fifty per cent chance of an unnecessary bilateral mastectomy represents a greater harm than some degree of psychological distress.

Utilitarianism strongly favours disclosure of the result

This is so merely when one considers Jane having a bilateral mastectomy. If one also adds the harm of removal of both her ovaries (the risks to life and health of the operation, the problems of long-term hormone replacement, the inability to have further children, etc.), there is an even more overwhelming case in favour of disclosure.

What kind of policy would utilitarians support on the disclosure of genetic test results to other family members? The geneticist says 'We feel we cannot approach people directly who have not been referred to us.' In general, most people would want to help their family members. The most cost-efficient policy is likely to be to encourage patients to inform their family members, as the current practice suggests. However, in those rare circumstances in which a patient refuses to inform a family member who is at grave risk, the geneticist should inform the family member directly. So the policy should be one of encouraging voluntary disclosure but in special circumstances doctors should disclose information directly to family members with an interest in it.

The geneticist also states that some centres require that patients consent to disclosure of the result to other family members as a precondition for testing. Utilitarians would support this if this policy had greater benefits overall than a policy of encouragement of voluntary disclosure with exceptional involuntary disclosure. Thus, which policy is better is an empirical issue for utilitarians. If significant numbers of people choose not to have testing if disclosure is a precondition, with harm to both themselves and their family members, then utilitarians would be against such a policy. If, on the other hand, few decided against testing because of the precondition of disclosure, the transparency of such a policy and the more fully informed consent that would follow would speak in its favour.

Egalitarian

Utiliarianism is egalitarian: no one's well-being counts more than anyone else's. The pauper's pain counts the same as the king's. As the father of utilitarianism, Jeremy Bentham put it: everybody to count for one, nobody for more than one.

Application

Everyone's well-being matters equally, including the well-being of Jane's husband and daughters. This means that we should take seriously the distress that they would experience if their wife or mother had a mastectomy or developed cancer. Utilitarians give great weight to the welfare of dependants in moral calculations.

Some would object that this feature of utilitarianism leads to unfairness. Why should the fact that Jane happens to have children who care about her mean that her well-being counts for more than Phyllis's well-being, because Phyllis has no dependants? However, in many cases in medicine, the interests of the family or other siblings do figure in decision-making. And if a mother has to provide for her children, many think this is a relevant consideration. This is a complex issue, which we cannot pursue here.

More straightforwardly, the interests of Jane's daughters in testing themselves and making the same kinds of decisions as Jane is now facing matter equally to the utilitarian. Without disclosure of Phyllis's result, then in order for Jane's daughters to be tested, it would be necessary for Jane to develop breast cancer. Otherwise there would be no way of giving a definitive diagnosis of which breast cancer gene is in the family. If Jane has a prophylactic mastectomy, both her daughters will be in the same situation as her – no way of accessing a predictive test. If they chose under this uncertainty to have a prophylactic mastectomy anyway, it is possible that three rather than one unnecessary bilateral mastectomy would have occurred. This is a disaster and counts heavily, at least for the utilitarian, in favour of disclosure. In short, and very roughly, for the utilitarian, this is not the conflict between the interests of Phyllis and Jane, but the conflict between the interests of Phyllis and three Janes.

Utilitarians also consider the impact of decisions on others in society. For utilitarians, the cost to society of healthcare for someone with breast cancer that could have been avoided is important. Indeed, even the resource cost of an unnecessary operation – in this case a bilateral mastectomy – is a moral consideration. Since disclosing the result will tend to promote Jane's health, and lower usage of the healthcare system, this will liberate more resources for the healthcare of others. Thus there are indirect benefits to others in society from disclosure. Utilitarianism sits very comfortably with a concern for public health and with the concern of health economists to use limited healthcare resources as efficiently as possible.

Utilitarianism is one member of a family of moral theories called consequentialism. The central tenet of consequentialism is that an action is right if, and only if, it promotes the best consequences. According to utilitarians, it is only the consequences for well-being that matter ('welfarism'). There are several versions of utilitarianism corresponding to how well-being is defined. There are three theories of well-being: hedonistic; desire-fulfilment; and objective list (Parfit 1984, Griffin 1986).

What is well-being?

Hedonistic utilitarianism

The classical utilitarians Jeremy Bentham and John Stuart Mill were hedonistic utilitarians. According to hedonistic utilitarians, well-being consists in valuable mental states. The doctrine of hedonism as expounded by Bentham describes only one valuable mental state (happiness or pleasure) and one negative mental state (unhappiness or pain) (Bentham 1948).

Preference utilitarianism

Utilitarians such as R. M. Hare and Peter Singer define human well-being as 'the obtaining to a high or at least reasonable degree of a quality of life which on the whole a person wants, or prefers to have' (Hare 1998).

Ideal Utilitarianism

According to ideal utilitarians like G. E. Moore, what matters is not mere happiness or achieving what we want, but doing worthwhile things.

[C]ertain things are good or bad for people, whether or not these people want to have the good things or avoid the bad things. The good things might include moral goodness, rational activity, the development of one's abilities, having children and being a good parent, knowledge and the awareness of true beauty. The bad things might include being betrayed, manipulated, slandered, deceived, being deprived of liberty and dignity, and enjoying either sadistic pleasure, or aesthetic pleasure in what is in fact ugly. (Parfit 1984: 499)

Each of these theories has its strengths and weaknesses as an account of what is good for people. Derek Parfit has argued that what is good is a combination of all three of these elements:

We might then claim that what is best for people is a composite ... We might claim, for example, that what is good or bad for someone is to have knowledge, to be engaged in rational activity, to experience mutual love, and to be aware of beauty, while strongly wanting these things. On this view, each side in the disagreement saw only half of the truth. Each put forward as sufficient something that was only necessary. Pleasure with many other kinds of object has no value. And, if they are entirely devoid of pleasure, there is no value in knowledge, rational activity, love, or awareness of beauty. What is of value, or is good for someone, is to have both; to be engaged in these activities, and to be strongly wanting to be so engaged. (Parfit 1984: 502)

Application

How much Phyllis and Jane are harmed or benefited by the act of disclosing the information depends on how we conceive of harm and benefit. On a very narrow medical account of well-being as health, it seems that Jane has a much greater stake in whether or not the information is disclosed. It is she who risks breast cancer and the complications of an unnecessary mastectomy.

However, even on a narrow account of well-being, the issue is not as straightforward as it appears. If Phyllis would suffer significant psychological effects from the disclosure of her information, e.g. develop depression, then this adverse effect on her mental health has to be balanced against the benefits to Jane's health. However, it is unlikely that Phyllis would suffer such catastrophic effects as to compare with the benefits to Jane of avoiding cancer and avoiding the complications, pain and disfigurement of an unnecessary mastectomy.

This claim – that the benefits in promotion of Jane's well-being are greater than the harms to Phyllis – is likely to be true no matter which account of well-being is employed. For example, the psychological consequences of developing cancer or having an unnecessary mastectomy are likely to be significantly greater, by orders of magnitude, than the consequences of having information about one's genetic status disclosed to a relative. Hedonistic utilitarianism supports disclosure.

Similarly, the strength of the preference to avoid cancer and an unnecessary mastectomy is likely to be significantly stronger than a preference to avoid disclosure. Preference utilitarianism supports disclosure.

Finally, according to ideal utilitarianism, there will be many benefits to disclosure. Jane will know that truth and knowledge are valuable in themselves. Also, this knowledge will allow Jane to plan her life more effectively. Avoiding cancer and unnecessary mastectomies will promote her life in many ways, e.g. by allowing positive relations with her husband and children. Some of the harms and benefits of genetic testing are outlined in Box 8.1 (after Savulescu 2002).

Box 8.1 Harms and benefits of predictive genetic testing for cancer

Potential harms
Development of a perception that the person is 'ill' with negative attitudes towards that person
Low self-esteem
Serious psychological maladjustment, even perhaps depression and suicide
Guilt
Impaired marital prospects
Disturbance of family relationships
Social discrimination, including future employment and insurance discrimination

Potential benefits
Prophylactic medical interventions
Minimises the possibility of serious psychological maladjustment later in life induced by late discovery of status

Decreased anxiety

Decreased uncertainty about the future

More realistic life choices, including more accurate reproductive, career, financial and health planning

Elimination of risk

More openness about genetic conditions within the family and society in general

Opportunity to use genetic testing in reproduction (prenatal or pre-implantation genetic diagnosis) to ensure offspring do not carry mutation

Act- versus rule-utilitarianism

There are two kinds of utilitarianism. According to act-utilitarianism, the right act is that particular act which promotes well-being to the greatest degree. According to rule-utilitarianism we should act according to rules (or laws), the adherence to which will most promote human well-being over time. We will discuss act-utilitarianism.

However, it is worth briefly discussing rule-utilitarianism. It is often argued that rule utilitarians would support always obeying rules such as respecting confidentiality. By always respecting confidentiality, doctors encourage patients to trust them and so disclose confidential information. If the rule is broken, patients will lose faith in their doctors with disastrous consequences of future patients failing to disclose vital confidential information relevant to their own diagnosis.

This, however, is a very narrow reading of rule-utilitarianism; rules can be complex. For example, always respect confidentiality except when there is a life-threatening risk to a family member of protecting confidentiality. Such rules may maximally promote well-being over time and not threaten trust in doctors. Most people, after all, want to help their family.

The legal basis for medical confidentiality is a form of this complex rule-utilitarianism. A doctor's legal obligation of confidentiality is a public, not a private, interest. It is for this reason that the obligation of confidentiality is not absolute. When a doctor breaches confidentiality, the law asks: is the balance of public interests in favour of breaching confidentiality or of maintaining it (Hope *et al.* 2003)? There are some examples where the law judges that it is in the public interest to require breach of confidentiality and other instances where it permits it. See Box 8.2 (after Hope *et al.* 2003).

Box 8.2 English law and breaching confidentiality

When doctors must breach confidentiality (to specific authorities only)
Notifiable diseases
Drug addiction
Termination of pregnancy
Births
Deaths
To police, on request: name and address of driver of vehicle who is alleged
 to be guilty of offence under Road Traffic Act (1988)
Search warrant signed by circuit judge
Under court orders

When doctors have discretion
Sharing information with other members of healthcare team in the inter-
 ests of the patient
Patient continuing to drive who is not medically fit to do so (NB The
 GMC now advises doctors to inform the DVLA medical officer)
When third party at significant risk of harm (e.g. spouse of HIV-positive
 person)

If the law and rule-utilitarianism both allow the breach of confidentiality in these circumstances, they would seem to allow disclosure in the current case since Jane's interest in the information is significant as there is a serious and direct risk of harm to her. Indeed, in the USA, patients have successfully sued doctors for failing to disclose confidential genetic information from other family members relating to risk of bowel cancer to them.

Utilitarianism and lying

The practices of promise keeping and telling the truth both generally promote well-being. Utilitarians strongly support social sanctions against lying. The geneticist in this case raises the possibility of 'fudging the issue', which was not possible in this case but may be possible in others. If 'fudging the issue' or lying in an exceptional circumstance did not have serious social consequences (eroding trust in doctors, etc.), and produced great good, the utilitarians would support fudging or even lying. Utilitarians famously hold that if you were hiding a Jewish person under your roof in the Second World War and a Nazi came to search your house, you should lie when he questions you about your relations with Jewish people.

Other features of utilitarianism

Decisions about right action require empirical evidence, including knowledge of the details (context) of a particular situation and of all alternative courses of action

In order to decide which action is right, we require information about what is likely to happen to people, now and in the future, as a result of the various alternative actions. Utilitarians also estimate how likely each outcome is to occur. The right action is the action that is most likely to have the best consequences. The goodness or badness of an outcome has to be balanced against how likely or unlikely that outcome is to occur. The mere existence of a chance that some action that is highly likely to have very good consequences for people might have some very small chance of causing a catastrophe is not sufficient to establish that the action is wrong – the action might be right if the chances of the good outcomes are sufficiently high, the good is sufficiently great and the chance of catastrophe sufficiently small.

For utilitarians, then, we must make our decisions on the best information available. But since we can never know the truth, we can never be absolutely certain, then we cannot demand that we know for certain which is the best course of action before proceeding. According to utilitarians, we should gather the best empirical evidence about the success rates of mastectomy, the cure rates for cancer, the psychological consequences of all courses of action, the effectiveness of the interventions for these and so on, but then we must make a decision about which course of action is likely to have the best overall consequences for all concerned. Utilitarianism thus sits very comfortably alongside evidence-based medicine.

Utilitarians also ask: what are the likely consequences of the action in this *particular* situation? Thus it is not sufficient to have a general knowledge of the psychological and sociological consequences of actions: in evaluating an act we must take account of specific details if they are available. For example, in order to evaluate whether killing a human being is wrong, utilitarians would want to know whether the killing of innocent people would be prevented, how many innocent lives would be saved and what consequences such a killing would have for law and order in society.

Sometimes this requirement for empirical evidence is used against utilitarians. How can we know which is the best course of action if we lack so much relevant information? For example, we simply do not know and have scarce sociological or psychological data on the effects of breaching confidentiality on the trust in doctors and the likely health consequences of any breach of trust on future patients.

There are several responses to this objection. First, such historical, socio-logical or psychological data, which are relevant to this issue, should be used. Often, we can gain some (rough) idea about the consequences of such a policy from other relevant policies. For example, there is a number of legally mandatory disclosures of medical information (see above). We can learn lessons from these social experiments. The requirement for some breaches of confidentiality does not seem to have disastrous consequences. Secondly, we have to decide on the basis of what information we have. Even if all existing evidence is weak, then utilitarianism still requires that we make a decision on the basis of it.

Alternatives

Utilitarians are concerned to evaluate the consequences of *all* available alter-native courses of action. We should ask: are there any other alternatives that we have not considered? So far we have considered the alternatives of:
1. disclosing the result:
   - Jane has a bilateral mastectomy if positive;
   - Jane does not have a bilateral mastectomy if negative.
2. not disclosing the result:
   - Jane has a bilateral mastectomy.
There is another alternative:
   - not disclosing the result and Jane does not have a prophylactic mas-tectomy but rather has aggressive screening for early breast cancer.

Application

The geneticist says:

It's true that there is not yet any research evidence that clearly shows that women who are likely to have one of these dominant breast-cancer genes should have prophylactic bilateral mastectomies recommended to them. But there *is* accumulating evidence that the lifetime risk of cancer following such an operation is significantly reduced; short-term follow-up studies of these women have shown that the cancer incidence is much lower in these women than in the same-risk women who are just screened regularly. However, there are not yet any data that suggest the *mortality* from breast cancer is reduced if these women have such an operation. Such data may never be collected, ... anecdotally since women may either want or not want such a major operation based more on their family's experience rather than on a risk figure which we provide for them.

When women have seen many women members of their family die from breast cancer, I think it not unreasonable to discuss such an operation as there is enough evidence to suggest it is *likely* to be of benefit. If there was absolutely clear evidence of benefit then it would be easier to argue that breaking Phyllis's confidentiality is justified in order to prevent serious harm, i.e. an unnecessary major operation.

Utilitarianism is a very practical theory. We should understand what all the relevant available alternatives are, gather the best available evidence on what the consequences of each of these are and, how likely each of these consequences are, and then we can make a decision based on this of what, on the balance of probabilities on the available evidence, is likely to have the best outcome.

Scientific evidence is very important for the utilitarian to decide which is the best course of action. In some cases, utilitarianism requires that we carry out good scientific research to gather evidence that will help us to decide which is the best course. But in the absence of, or prior to, such scientific research, utilitarianism requires that we make a decision now about what is the best course.

In some circumstances, it may be most prudent to wait until the evidence is available. For example, if it were very unclear that prophylactic mastectomy would confer any benefits, and a large trial of prophylactic mastectomy would be completed in one year, it may be prudent for Jane to wait a year for these results.

Intentional omissions are morally equivalent to intentional acts

For utilitarians, deciding to do nothing is one course of action. Its consequences have to be compared to the consequences of acting in other ways. To fail to promote a person's well-being is morally equivalent to harming that person. So the doctor cannot escape responsibility by claiming that he or she will do nothing in this case and not disclose the result. To decide not to disclose the result is an action, the consequences of which we are responsible for.

Utilitarianism is demanding

As utilitarians consider omissions to be equivalent to acts, utilitarianism is a very demanding moral theory – some say too demanding. It implies that intentionally to fail to save someone's life is the same as killing them. For example, failing to send ten pounds a month that would save a child's life in a developing country is morally equivalent to killing that child. And this applies to another ten pounds that could save another child. And so on until virtually all our wage is consumed in saving people's lives. Utilitarianism seems to require endless self-sacrifice provided that the benefits to others outweigh (even slightly) the losses to us.

An infamous example is John Harris's 'The survival lottery':

[E]veryone is given a sort of lottery number. Whenever doctors have two or more dying patients who could be saved by transplants, and no suitable organs . . . they ask a central computer to supply a suitable donor. The computer will then pick the number of a suitable donor at random and he will be killed so that the lives of the two more others may be saved . . . [E]ven taking into account the loss of the lives of donors, the numbers of untimely deaths each year might be dramatically reduced, so much so that everyone's chance of living to a ripe old age might be increased. (Harris 2001)

According to utilitarians, there is nothing wrong with killing an innocent person (indeed, it may be morally required) if it promotes well-being overall. This seems highly counter-intuitive.

This objection can, however, be turned on its head. Those who believe that there is absolute prohibition on killing innocent people also face a problem. Imagine that the only way to prevent the *certain* release of chemical and biological weapons, which will cause the deaths of millions of innocent people, is to invade a country and overthrow the regime, killing hundreds of innocent people. According to utilitarians, such an action might be justified if the certainty of harm were sufficiently high and the number of innocent deaths caused by invasion sufficiently low. According to those who believe we can never intentionally kill the innocent, such actions could never be justified.

Another response is that many alternative moral theories are too undemanding. Often, morality is constructed to fit intuitions about everyday practice. Such theories simply serve to promulgate the status quo, which is often based on bias, prejudice or arbitrary cultural practice. Utilitarianism is based on an uncontroversial moral consideration: human well-being. Utilitarianism serves to challenge any practice that fails to promote human well-being.

Utilitarianism is a theory that is 'spatially and temporally neutral'

Well-being matters equally, whatever its spatio-temporal location. A person's suffering is equally important whether it occurs now or in the future, here or in Afghanistan. Even effects several generations later matter equally.

Application

Utilitarianism gives equal weight to the interests of future generations. According to utilitarians, it is better if children are born without the gene for breast cancer (or other deleterious genes) because these genes reduce the opportunities to have the best and longest life. So utilitarians would strongly favour disclosure because it would not only allow Jane to test herself but also allow her to use the test if she were to become pregnant again, in order to see whether her unborn child possessed one of these genes. While it does not sound like Jane is considering having more children from the story (indeed whether she can have more children), this issue is certainly relevant to her daughters.

Indeed, if the gene were identified in the family, this would give Jane's daughters at least two choices if they were considering having a family of their own. First, they could become pregnant and use prenatal testing at about ten weeks of pregnancy to see if their child had the gene. If it did, they could choose to terminate the pregnancy and become pregnant again in an attempt to have a child who does not have this mutation.

Second, they could use in-vitro fertilisation to produce a number of embryos. These embryos could be subjected to genetic testing using pre-implantation genetic diagnosis. This would identify disease-free embryos which could then be transferred.

According to utilitarians, if a couple are going to have a fixed number of children, e.g. two, then they should have two children without genetic mutations using either of these technologies. Not only do they believe that it is right to use such genetic testing but that it is wrong not to use genetic testing in reproduction.

In this case, Jane's interest in the genetic information is personal – she is contemplating prophylactic surgery. In other cases in genetics, Jane's interest will purely be to inform her reproductive decision-making. Thus a woman may be a carrier of a genetic condition and herself be unaffected but at risk of having a child with serious genetic condition, e.g. muscular dystrophy. A situation may arise similar to the case under discussion in which a family member is aware of a genetic mutation but this woman is unaware of it. The only relevance of the information would be to enable this woman to have preimplantation genetic diagnosis or prenatal testing to ensure she does not have a child affected by the mutation. Utilitarians see such testing as right and morally required because it will result in a healthy rather than unhealthy child. Not only is the well-being of the child higher, but the parents are likely to have a less difficult time and the costs of healthcare will be lower. Utilitarians would favour disclosure in such situations.

Utilitarianism and personal autonomy

'Autonomy' comes from the Greek *autos* and *nomos* meaning self-rule. It refers to the capacity of most human beings to form their own idea of what is good for them and how they should lead their own lives. Respect for autonomy, including respect for people's own choices about their lives, is one of the cornerstone principles of medical ethics. Respect for confidentiality is derivative from respect for autonomy. In its concern to promote human well-being, utilitarianism may seem to give insufficient importance to people's autonomy. Utilitarians can be caricatured as totalitarians trampling the freedom of the individual.

Utilitarians, however, give great weight to personal autonomy. The father of liberalism, John Stuart Mill, who wrote the classic defence of personal autonomy entitled *On Liberty*, was a hedonistic utilitarian. Mill argued that in general, people's well-being is best promoted by allowing people freedom to construct their own original existence, to discover what kind of life is best for themselves:

Individuality is the same thing with development, and . . . it is only the cultivation of individuality which produces, or can produce, well-developed humans . . . (Mill 1910: 121)

This quote comes from the chapter from *On Liberty* entitled 'Of individuality, as one of the elements of well-being.' Mill clearly believes that individuality is one of the goods of life. Mill calls 'inviduality' what we call 'autonomy.' Mill gives great importance to autonomy rather than living according to prevailing custom or the judgements of others:

I have said that it is important to give the freest scope possible to uncustomary things, in order that it may appear in time which of these *are fit to be converted into customs*. But independence of action, and disregard of custom, are not solely deserving of encouragement for the chance they afford that better modes of action, and customs more worthy of general adoption, may be struck out; nor is it only persons of decided mental superiority who have a just claim to carry on their lives in their own way. There is no reason that all human existence should be constructed on some one or small number of patterns. *If a person possesses any tolerable amount of common sense and experience, his own mode of laying out his existence is the best, not because it is the best in itself, but because it is his own mode.* [my italics] (Mill 1910: 125)

The GP's claim – 'I think she should just have regular screens' – is wrong. For the utilitarian, Jane should decide for herself whether the benefits of mastectomy outweigh the risks. Moreover, on any account of well-being (hedonistic, desire-fulfilment, or objective list) she will be best placed to decide whether the consequences of mastectomy promote her well-being. She will know how it will affect her mental state, how strongly she desires it and how it will affect her capacity to engage in worthwhile activities. The GP is paternalistic and his paternalism is based on false assessments of Jane's well-being.

Utilitarians thus give great importance to obtaining properly informed consent for medical procedures because this is one way to respect people's autonomy.

The oncologist alludes to the fact that genetic tests have implications for other family members. He raises the issue of whether doctors should seek consent from family members before performing a genetic test on a patient. He argues that they should not. While utilitarians place great weight on respect for personal autonomy, they would not generally support a practice of obtaining consent from other family members before performing a test. The costs of such a practice are likely to be high and the benefits small. In the vast majority of cases, there are not conflicts between family members as in this case, and in the minority, the individual clinician should make a judgement about what is best for all concerned on a case-by-case basis.

Although the utilitarian gives great importance to liberty and autonomy, when people's life plans conflict and others are harmed by our choices, then we should perform that action which promotes well-being most. Then we must make an assessment of whose well-being is most affected. When choices have serious life-threatening implications for others, as in this case, then liberty can be constrained.

Utilitarianism is not retributive

According to retributive theories of justice, justice should be sensitive to and correct past wrongs. The classic formulation of this is 'an eye for an eye'. Utilitarianism does not consider past wrongs per se. For the utilitarian, the fact that someone has been wronged in the past does increase their claim. What matters is well-being and we should do whatever will maximise well-being now and in the future.

Phyllis attempts to appeal to retributive considerations when she says 'I told the doctor how I'd nursed my mother and my sister when they were dying. Both didn't thank me for it. My sister and I had a huge row about money just before she died – it was dreadful. I wasn't even mentioned in her will and the family completely ignored me afterwards. I don't feel I owe them anything.' Whether or not Phyllis was actually wronged, these considerations are irrelevant to the utilitarian. We should not harm Jane and her daughters even if Phyllis was wronged in the past.

There may be another wrong in this case. The oncologist did not inform Phyllis of many of the consequences of the genetic test, including the consequences for her family members. The oncologist may not have obtained properly informed consent for the test. Even if this were the case, and Phyllis were wronged, this would not be a reason to withhold the information that may prevent serious harm to Jane and her daughters. Utilitarians believe we should use such 'tainted' data if they promote people's well-being. (Utilitarians would, of course, be in favour of compensating individuals who had been harmed by not giving properly informed consent as this will both promote their well-being and the practice of respecting personal autonomy by obtaining informed consent, which promotes well-being overall.)

Testing children

Imagine that it turns out that Jane does carry the breast-cancer gene. One of the major ethical issues in clinical genetics is predictive genetic testing of children. Should we test Jane's daughters?

If Jane's daughters are competent adolescents then there are good reasons to leave the decision to them (Robertson and Savulescu 2001, Savulescu 2001). But what if the children are younger – should we test them before they are able to decide for themselves?

For the utilitarian, whether or not they should be tested depends on whether they will be better off by being tested now. Since none of the medical interventions available would be employed during childhood, many geneticists would be against testing young children. The benefits of waiting are that the individual can make the decision for herself, and this kind of liberty has great value for utilitarians. However, if there are benefits of early testing in terms of earlier and more effective psychological adaptation and development of more realistic life plans, then these must be considered. The issue is not straightforward for the utilitarian and will depend on scientific evidence about the effects of predictive genetic testing in children (Robertson and Savulescu 2001, Savulescu 2001).

Summary

In summary, utilitarians would strongly favour the disclosure of this result for the following reasons:
1. the benefits to Jane's well-being greatly outweigh the harm to Phyllis's well-being of disclosure;
2. Jane's daughters themselves can be tested, which will promote their well-being;
3. there are benefits to the well-being of Jane's family;
4. testing would allow Jane or her children to use prenatal or preimplantation genetic testing to ensure that they do not have children with the same mutations;
5. there are benefits to society in the form of lower healthcare costs.

REFERENCES

Bentham, J. (1948). *The Principles of Morals and Legislation*. New York: Hafner. [Originally published 1789.]

Griffin, J. (1986). *Well-Being*. Oxford: Clarendon Press.

Hare, R. M. (1998). A utilitarian approach. In H. Kuhse and P. Singer, eds., *A Companion to Bioethics*. Oxford: Blackwell, 80–5.

Harris, J. (2001). The survival lottery. In J. Harris, ed., *Bioethics*. Oxford: Oxford University Press, 300–15.

Hope, T., Savulescu, J. and Hendrick, J. (2003). *Medical Ethics and Law: The Core Curriculam*. Edinburgh: Churchill Livingstone.

Mill, J. S. (1910). *On Liberty*. London: J. M. Dent and Sons. [Originally published 1859.]

Parfit, D. (1984). *Reasons and Persons*. Oxford: Clarendon Press, 493–502.

Robertson, R. and Savulescu, J. (2001). Is there a case in favour of predictive testing of children? *Bioethics*, **15**, 1526–49.

Savulescu, J. (2001). Predictive genetic testing in children. *Med J Australia*, **175**, 379–81.

(2003). Bioethics: utilitarianism. In D. Cooper, ed., *Nature Encylopaedia of the Human Genome, Volume 1*. London: Nature Publishing Group, 288–95.

9

A feminist care-ethics approach to genetics

Marian Verkerk

Feminist care-ethics makes a difference when analysing and discussing healthcare issues. As a specific moral perspective it frames moral questions in healthcare in terms of responsibilities and is concerned more about the dangers of *abandonment* than the dangers of *interference*. The care perspective also invites us to re-examine and re-evaluate current conceptions of autonomy and moral relationships. In this chapter I shall try to show that care-ethics, as a relational ethics, makes a difference in the moral reading of problems arising in the use of genetics. In arguing this, I will start by presenting the main characteristics of care-ethics. I will then go on to discuss the issue of whether care-ethics can be seen as a *feminist* ethical perspective. In the final part of the chapter I will show how care ethics can make a difference to the discussion of ethical issues in genetics. In particular, I shall concentrate on the tension between responsibility toward others and the value of personal autonomy.

Care ethics

In 1982, Carol Gilligan published *In a Different Voice*, in which she put forward the thesis that a so-called ethics of justice gives only a partial voice to the moral experiences of men and especially of women. An ethics of justice, needs to be complemented by an ethics of care that is capable of articulating the moral values of nurturing and caring. In developing this care perspective Gilligan challenged the idea that abstract and universalistic moral reasoning was the best way of thinking about moral problems.[1] She proposes an alternative perspective in which particularities, relationships and continued connection are emphasised. In proposing this alternative moral perspective, Gilligan did not state that an ethics of care is exclusively women's or feminine morality, but she did suggest that women more than men tended to think in those moral terms.

Case Analysis in Clinical Ethics, ed. Richard Ashcroft, Anneke Lucassen, Michael Parker, Marian Verkerk, Guy Widdershoven. Published by Cambridge University Press.

Gilligan's work as a psychologist has been further developed by feminist ethicists and philosophers. Nell Nodding's *Caring: A Feminine Approach to Ethics and Moral Education* and Virginia Held's *Feminist Morality* are well-known examples of care-ethics approaches (Noddings 1984, Held 1993).

Although there are already many versions of care ethics, which differ sometimes in substantial ways, all of them at least contain the two following assumptions:

1. the main characteristic of human existence is relationality; and
2. moral reasoning is characterised by moral sensitivity, attentiveness and connectedness.

The first characteristic expresses an anthropological and ontological view about human existence. Care ethicists criticise the central role that the notion of self-sufficient independence tends to play in moral thinking in Western culture. This notion functions both descriptively and prescriptively to promote a particular conception of human nature and of the telos of human life. On this view, human beings are seen as capable of leading self-sufficient, isolated and independent lives. From this premise is drawn the prescriptive conclusion that the goal of human life is the realisation of self-sufficiency and individuality. Lorraine Code explains this as:

Autonomous man is – and should be – self-sufficient, independent and self-reliant, a self-realizing individual who directs his efforts towards maximizing his personal gains. His independence is under constant threat from other (equally self-serving) individuals: hence he devises rules to protect himself from intrusion. Talk of rights, rational self-interest, expedience and efficiency permeates his moral, social and political discourse. (Code 1991)

In opposition to this notion, care ethics proposes a view of human existence that is characterised as relational and interdependent. For instance, in describing the self, Held presents a view of the human self that seems to be the opposite of the autonomous self as described above:

The self . . . is seen as having both a need for recognition and a need to understand the other, and these needs are seen as compatible. They are created in the context of mother–child interaction and are satisfied in a mutually empathetic relationship . . . Both give and take in a way that not only contributes to the satisfaction of their needs as individuals but also affirms the 'larger relational unit' they compose. Maintaining this larger relational unit then becomes a goal and maturity is seen not in terms of individual autonomy but in terms of competence in creating and sustaining relations of empathy and mutual intersubjectivity. (Held 1993)

The second characteristic of care ethics that I mentioned involves requirements about what constitutes adequate moral reasoning. The claim is that instead of the skill of abstraction, a skill of an attunement to difference should be developed in moral reasoning. The requirements of universality and impartiality in the so-called ethics of justice overlook the importance of partiality, context and relational bonds in moral life (Wolf 1996). In care ethics, respecting a person does not involve valuing and treating her as case of generic personhood, but more as the whole, and concrete, particular person she is. More emphasis should be laid on a moral ideal of *attention* as a commitment to attend all aspects of the irreducible particularity of individual human persons in their concrete contexts. Attention, contextual and narrative appreciation, and communication are considered to be key elements of moral deliberation.

Although care ethics has largely been developed by feminist theorists, the ideas of care ethics appear elsewhere in the history of philosophy and ethics (Reich 1995). For instance, Paul Ricoeur understands care as solicitude in a fundamental anthropological terms. In his book *Oneself as Another*, he writes about 'care' as 'solicitude':

Our self is inseparable with the recognition of fragility and mortality of human existence. In true sympathy, the self, whose power of acting is at the start greater than that of its other, finds itself affected by all that the suffering others offers to it in return. This is perhaps the supreme test of solicitude, when unequal power finds compensation in an authentic reciprocity in exchange, which, in the hour of agony, finds refuge in the shared whisper of voices or the feeble embrace of clasped hands. (Ricoeur 1992)

We come across this tone of relationality and of the fragility of human existence again in the definitions of care provided by Joan Tronto and Bernice Fisher:

Caring is to be viewed as a species activity that includes everything that we do to maintain, continue, and repair our 'world' so that we can live in it as well as possible. That world includes our bodies, our selves, and our environment, all of which we seek to interweave in a complex, life-sustaining web. (Tronto 1993)

Care, as a specific moral sentiment, was also apparent in the history of philosophy and ethics long before this. Adam Smith, David Hume and Joseph Butler make room for sentiments such as sympathy and benevolence in moral reasoning. There is a difference, however, between these views and the ethics of care. With this view, care is not to be understood in terms of sympathy for our fellow human being, but is directed to the particularity of the other. In care we recognise and respect the other in her particularity, as the whole and concretely particular person she is, with her own needs, desires and opportunities, with her own history and her own view of life.

Despite the aforementioned exceptions, the history of philosophy and ethics does not contain many examples in which care is treated as an important concept. Justice, freedom and equality play a far more important role in this history. It is not an exaggeration to say that care, loyalty and friendship as important moral concepts have tended to be neglected or marginalised in the ethical, political and philosophical discourses of our Western culture.

The care perspective can be roughly summarised as the perspective aimed at developing ways of living well in concrete relationships with others, responding to their needs and building up a joint life. It thereby underlines the importance of connection and attachment.

The question remains, however, of whether or not care ethics should be seen as a full-blown ethical theory and if so, what kind of ethical theory it is. For some, care ethics is a version of virtue ethics; for others care ethics is best thought of as a normative theory of right action in which the principle of care is the main principle. In the latter case, it remains to be seen in what way the principle of care differs from other principles such as beneficence or fidelity. In the former case – that care ethics is a form of virtue ethics – there is also a need to explain what kind of virtue care is and how it distinguishes itself from virtues such as love and compassion (Veatch 1998).

Instead of presenting care ethics as a virtue ethics or as a normative theory of right action, I shall take a different route. Following Margaret Olivia Little, I will understand care ethics as a moral *perspective* or *orientation* to the moral world. The care perspective is thereby defined in terms of *emphases of concern and discernment* (to notice and worry more, say, about the dangers of abandonment rather than the dangers of interference), *habits and proclivities of interpretation* (the proclivity, say, to read *the* moral question presented by a situation in terms of responsibilities rather than rights) and *selectivity of skills* (to have developed, say, an attunement to difference than an ease of abstraction) (Little 1998). Little emphasises the idea that care ethics is a stance from which to carry out theory, rather than as constituting a ready-made theory in its own right. Although this will sound to some as too modest a claim on behalf of care ethics, I think that Little makes an important point here. For instance, care ethics has been criticised both because its claims are either too broad or too narrow. In claiming that people should care for each other, it urges either expansive obligations to the world at large or it remains too parochial in its responsibilities. But as Little points out, 'the truth is that the care orientation in and of itself does not claim either.' What we should do, she suggests, is examine the results of theorising *from the lens* of this care orientation and see what views emerge about the claims of 'strangers' and 'intimates' (Little 1998: 204). And even if reflections through the lens of care ethics lead to policies similar to those offered by other ethical and non-feminist approaches, the differences in approach still matter through influencing what precedent one takes oneself to have set, what dangers one is alerted to watch for, and what would later count as good reasons to abandon or rethink the policy. For instance, trust, loyalty, friendship and caring as important moral concepts tend to be neglected or marginalised in other mainstream ethical discourses. Furthermore, concepts such as respect take on a different meaning within the care perspective. For instance, Robin Dillon has developed a care perspective based on the notion of respect, in which respect for a person involves valuing and treating her not as a case of generic personhood but as the whole and concretely particular person she is (Dillon 1992).

Is care ethics a feminist ethics?

Rosemary Tong once distinguished at least three feminist approaches to ethics, ignoring in so doing all kinds of intermediate forms: there is, she argued, a liberal, a radical and a cultural version of feminist ethics (Tong 1996). All three approaches share two assumptions that Alison Jagger once identified in feminist theory: 'the moral experience of women is worthy of respect and the subordination of women is morally wrong' (Jaggar 1989). On the other hand, each of the different approaches identified by Tong differs in their answer to the question of how to give moral voice to women and how to end the subordination of women. The liberal feminist is mainly committed to equal opportunities for women and men in the public and private spheres. The radical feminist approach stresses the women's reproductive roles and responsibilities, as well as the ideal of compulsory heterosexuality as the fundamental causes of women's oppression by men (Rich 1980). Cultural feminists emphasise the value of nurturing and caring as human values, which have been neglected in male-dominated ethical theory so far. To the extent that those values have played a role in theory and practice, they have been strictly seen as traditionally female values. By positively valuing the activity of caring and responsibility of care, care ethics can be seen as a version of cultural feminism.

For some, it remains to be seen whether care ethics is a *feminist* theory at all. The ethic of care seems to validate skills and virtues traditionally associated with women and women's roles. This presents feminists with a dilemma. On the one hand, there is a vital need for an ethic that takes the experience of women seriously, and the ethic of care does just that, capturing certain features of our moral lives that other more standard approaches to morality underplay or ignore. On the other hand, care ethics threatens to support and sustain the subordinate status of women in society, contributing to the exploitation and denigration of women with which feminist ethics is more broadly concerned. The distribution of caring falls disproportionately to women in our society, and even more so to women who are poor and non-white. Research also shows that responsibility for family health falls disproportionately to women in Western society. By virtue of both reproductive capacity and social positioning, the role of family caregivers has traditionally fallen to women. It seems that women bear more of the responsibility for monitoring health issues in families than men. Traditional practices of care in which care was seen as solely a 'women's practice' have undermined the personal autonomy of women themselves. For a long time women have been socialised to curb their ambitions and to identify themselves with the goals of others, neglecting their own. Connected with this, the other fact that caring work is very much socially devalued in society only makes the situation for women worse.

Care ethics is also sometimes criticised because the very structure of the caring relationship would seem to lead to the marginalisation of those who are dependent and in need of help. It would seem to threaten an oppressive paternalism. Anita Silvers had put this criticism in the following words:

Helping relationships are voluntary, but asymmetrically so. Help-givers choose how they are willing to help, but help-takers cannot choose how they will be helped, for in choosing to reject proffered help one withdraws oneself from being helped as well as from being in a helping relationship. To relate to others primarily by being helped by them, then, implies subordination of one's choices to one's caretakers, at least insofar as one remains in the state of being helped. (Silvers 1995)

Hoagland and Tong also warn us about the arbitrary and abusive uses of caretaker power. We need to be on our guard against the potential for cruel or disabling exercises of maternal authority and discretionary leeway (Hoagland 1990).

And so, if it is shown that the above threats are real, feminists may feel obliged to repudiate the approach (Carse and Lindemann Nelson 1996). In order to present care ethics not merely as a feminine but as a feminist ethics two criticisms need to be addressed:

- the exploitation and self-effacement of the care-giver; and
- the oppression of the care-receiver.

The caring relationship

I will answer these criticisms by exploring the nature of the caring relationship itself.

Care ethicists have been aware of the dangers of vicarious identification, projection and carers' desires to control those for whom they care, and the dangers of maintaining others in a state of dependence. Genuine sensitivity and attentiveness have therefore been put forward as crucial to achieving an understanding of the way others see and experience their needs and thus to the ability to care for them effectively. According to Joan Tronto, genuine attentiveness allows the caretaker to see through pseudo-needs and come to appreciate what the other really needs. Also Margaret Urban Walker states that:

... acuity of moral perception, especially as regards the interests and perspectives of people, must result from the exercise of many complex, learned, and indefinitely improvable skills of attention, communication and interpretation. (Walker 1991a)

Genuine attentiveness requires self-knowledge so that the caretaker does not transform the needs of the other into a projection of their own needs. A so-called 'care for the self' is therefore necessary (Hampton 1997). In stipulating the need for a care for the self, the care perspective differs from an impartialist or justice perspective. In this latter perspective, theoretical postulates such as the ideal observer, the disinterested judge, the archangel, the original position and the view from nowhere are designed to correct for the assumed bias of particular points of view (Jaggar 1995). Whereas impartialist perspectives of these kinds bracket or disregard the particular self in a certain way, care ethics points to appropriate motivations, attitudes, sensibilities and qualities of character which are thought indispensable to morally acute perception.

In addition to the need for a care for the self, caring intentions should also be validated through communication with those cared for. As Walker writes:

Asking, telling, repeating, mutually clarifying, mulling over, and checking back are the most dependable, accessible, and efficient devices for finding out how it is with others. (Walker 1991b)

The care ethics approach not only pays more attention to the moral qualities of the subject, but also conceptualises differently the relation between that subject and the object of her moral concern. Care ethics is personal and particularised in that both carers and those cared for regard each other as unique irreplaceable individuals. It is because of this that Dillon introduces the concept of 'care as respect' – recognising our power to make and unmake each other as persons and exercising this power wisely and carefully. As she says:

... care respect involves a determination to discover, forge, repair, and strengthen connections among persons in ways that benefit all of us. It joins individuals together in a community of mutual concern and mutual aid, through an appreciation of individuality and interdependence. (Dillon 1992)

Good caring involves a view of the caring relationship as an ongoing process and, what is more, caring relationships should also be viewed as embedded practices. Tronto states that care is a complex process that ultimately reflects structures of power and inequality. It is because of this that Tronto emphasised the need for a 'political argument' for an ethics of care (Tronto 1993). Within this political argument social practices that use care roles to exploit or oppress can be criticised. Caring relationships are only morally justified in situations in which there is an equality of access to care and equality in the distribution of care responsibilities. A feminist care ethics should therefore bring into the foreground the ways caring responsibilities are engendered and infused by power relations.

What implications does a feminist care ethics, as a moral orientation, have for questions relating to genetics? In answering this question, I will concentrate on the moral question of what responsibilities individuals should have to one another with respect to genetic knowledge and how the value of personal autonomy fits in.

Genetics and the need for a relational perspective

Laurence McCullough writes that the old infectious-disease model has been replaced by molecular medicine (McCullough 1998). This older model understood diseases in terms of foreign agents that cause disease. In so far as individuals carried moral obligations related to health, they had the obligation not to infect others. In contrast to the older infectious disease model, molecular medicine understands disease and health in terms of the interaction of genes and environment. The scientific explanation of health and disease in molecular medicine assumes not that we are isolated individuals at risk of alien invasions but that we are connected individuals. Genetic decision-making should therefore pay more attention to interpersonal dependencies in families. This aspect of relatedness is also implied in the way genetic data are viewed. Although genetic data must be obtained from individuals, they are not really individual data. Genetic data provide information not only about the individual from whom a sample is taken but also about related individuals. For McCullough this all implies that 'moral responsibilities of patients become a fundamental category – at least as fundamental as rights: perhaps when the interests of others are vitally at stake, more fundamental' (McCullough 1998).

In short, McCullough advocates a relational approach in analysing and tackling moral issues related to genetics. And I agree with him. Care ethics as an example of a relational approach can make a difference in the moral reading on genetics in at least three points.

First, the development of genetics brings the question of relationality in human existence to the fore. One of the main characteristics of hereditary diseases is that the information of one's genetic constitution will have consequences for one's kin: hereditary diseases are family diseases. The patient is not only an individual but also a member of a family and embedded in familial relationships. Care ethics with its emphasis on relationality and connectedness as the main characteristics of human existence can therefore be of use in analysing moral issues that arise from developments in the field of new genetics.[2]

Second, modern genetics invites us to address the question of what responsibilities individuals have to one another with respect to genetic knowledge. Care ethics is a moral orientation that frames moral questions in terms of what responsibilities we have to each other and toward ourselves, instead of posing moral questions in terms of conflicting moral rights. In thinking about our moral responsibilities in relation to issues of genetics, care ethics can give us important insights.

Third, an ethical approach to how to deal with the disclosure of genetic information seems to call for a broad sensitivity. This includes sensitivity to family dynamics, attention to the effects of social arrangements on moral understandings and experiences and respect for agency as lived. It seems, therefore, that the moral duty to disclose genetic information is something that cannot be abstractly assigned. Rather it is a duty that acquires meaning, is lived out and therefore can be evaluated only in the life context of particular individuals. A care-ethics approach with its emphasis on attention, and contextual and narrative appreciation as elements of moral deliberations is well suited to this task.

The care-ethics approach gives a different reading of the moral problems related to the case of Phyllis and Jane. In the presentation of the case, the moral problem is formulated as an issue where 'the clinician has to choose between preserving the confidentiality of one relative versus enhancing the autonomy of another by allowing them fully informed choices.' In other words, the moral problem is interpreted in terms of conflicting rights: the right to make an autonomous decision and the right to confidentiality. Those who regard confidentiality as sacrosanct would disregard Jane's interests rather than breach confidential information. The tested individual has a stronger claim to the information than other family members, so she ought not to be compelled to disclose the information. Conversely, there are those who claim that the importance of accurate information for someone's future plans should trump one's other right to confidentiality.

Instead of a moral reading in terms of conflicting rights, I will address the moral questions arising in this case in terms of what responsibilities individuals should have to one another with respect to genetic knowledge. Does Phyllis have a responsibility towards Jane, because Jane is family and vulnerable to the actions of Phyllis? Does this responsibility overrule the right of personal autonomy of Phyllis and her right not to be interfered with? In other words, what can we say about the tension between responsibility towards others, in particularly family and the value of personal autonomy?

Responsibility and the value of personal autonomy

At first sight, Phyllis would be unlikely to be very keen on the implications of a care-ethics approach, especially not with its emphasis on the value of relationality and its connected responsibilities. In fact, she is fed up with all these relations and feels that they have done her no good at all. As Phyllis said

'I told the doctor how I'd nursed my mother and my sister when they were dying. Neither of them thanked me for it. My sister and I had a huge row about money just before she died – it was dreadful. I wasn't even mentioned in her will and the family completely ignored me afterwards. I don't feel I owe them anything.' Phyllis does not feel any obligations towards her family. In fact, Phyllis takes the moral stance of not wanting to be interfered with. And who would want to blame her for that? She was the one who took care of her mother and sister and received nothing. Phyllis sacrificed her life for her family and had to forget all about her own personal self and life.

Both GPs of Jane and Phyllis seem to agree with Phyllis's reason not to disclose the test result. They said 'her main reasons are that she would feel blamed by the family and I think that it is reasonable'.

Whether Phyllis's reasons are indeed reasonable remains to be seen. But what seems to be true is that the simple fact that someone is related as family to someone is not enough reason to have an obligation towards him or her. Although family relationships count, the history of that relationship and the particulars of the relationships and situation also count in determining the moral weight of responsibilities and obligations that we have towards each other. Assigning responsibilities are only intelligible against a background of existing practices and its normative expectations, as Walker would say (Walker 1991a,b).

I will come back to the question of responsibility later. Meanwhile, there is a second issue to be raised: is it right to take Phyllis's wish not to be interfered with at face value? That is, is Phyllis's wish an autonomous wish at all?

Care ethics and autonomy

As we know, the idea of choice and autonomous decision-making is important in almost every bioethical reflection. So too in feminist theory, particularly in liberal feminism, the idea of free choice and autonomous decision-making is central to the empowerment of women. Nevertheless, it seems that in mainstream bioethics a particularly individualistic conception of autonomy tends to be adopted. As Rosemary Tong states it:

... within the deep structure of traditional ethics and bioethics, a creature known as the autonomous self, generally pictured as a biological male, and intent on maximizing his self-interest. (Tong 1996: 82)

The individual decision maker is idealised and non-embedded. Agents are not seen as emotional, irrational and embodied creatures and the options for choice are abstracted from complex social and cultural contexts. In this conception of personal autonomy, which motivates much healthcare practice, formal informed consent requirements are emphasised and the background conditions, in which choices are made, are ignored. The individual decision maker is regarded in isolation from significant relations with surrounding others.

In feminist care ethics, by contrast, a reconceptualisation of autonomy is proposed in which the social dimension of agency and selfhood is emphasised. This alternative conception is often called 'relational autonomy' (Mackenzie and Stoljar 2000).

In developing a relational account of autonomy, the idea of autonomy in terms of self-governance is not deserted. Rather, the overly individualistic account of human nature, which seems to underlie dominant conceptions of autonomy, is criticised. In the relational approach a richer account of the autonomous agent is developed. The self is an 'encumbered self', always already embedded in relationships with others and partly constituted by these relationships. According to Anne Donchin, relationships are of importance in developing autonomy in at least two senses. First, autonomy is not solely an individual enterprise but involves a dynamic balance among interdependent people tied to overlapping projects. The self-determining self is continually remaking itself in response to relationships that are seldom static. Interconnections continue to shape and define us throughout our lifetimes. Second, an appropriate respect for personal autonomy requires others to respond sensitively to the patient and help to restore and strengthen autonomy competencies (Donchin 2000).

Diana Meyers, for instance, suggests that we should think about autonomy as a *competency*, which, in its turn, is defined as a repertory of coordinated skills that enables a person to perform a specified task (Meyers 1989). These skills are used in concert in order to carry out a procedure that allows one to monitor one's conduct and determine whether or not it is in accordance with one's true self. An autonomous agent asks questions such as 'can I take responsibility for this or that action while retaining my self respect?' or 'could I bear to be the sort of person who can do that?' The true self that is consulted in this process is not to be understood as a true self in ontological terms, as a self that can be discovered by stripping back the layers of socialisation. Instead, the true self is dynamic, it is – as Meyers puts it – an evolving collocation of traits that emerges through the use of autonomy competency (Meyers 1989). The true self is an 'encumbered self', a self that is always already embedded in relationships with flesh and blood others and is partly constituted by these relations.

From the viewpoint of a relational account of autonomy, we could raise questions concerning whether Phyllis is autonomous in her decision-making. Phyllis says that she wants to be left alone, but does she really? Phyllis's self is constituted by the relationships in which she has been embedded. Her self is the result of disappointments. Phyllis would certainly feel differently, and would probably have decided differently, if she had felt respected by her family. The geneticist tells us that she has tried her hardest to negotiate with Phyllis and to persuade her of the potential benefit to unaffected relatives. She speaks of Phyllis as 'a sad and isolated lady who shouldn't be bullied into doing something she thinks will bring her harm.' It could be said that the geneticist has some doubt about taking the choice of Phyllis at face value and seeing Phyllis as an autonomous agent. One might go even further and argue that the present self of Phyllis is not the authentic one. Phyllis cannot be seen as an autonomous person as long as she experiences herself as degraded and worthless. Not only self-respect but also self-worth comprise necessary conditions for autonomy (Govier 1993, Benson 2000). What is more, an adequate normative identity and self-understanding, which makes valuing oneself a real possibility, is itself only possible in the context of loving relationships and through changing from a self-obsessive mode to one that centrally involves attentive care (Dillon 1992).

From a relational account of autonomy a less non-directive model of genetic counselling might be defended. Professionals in healthcare should help their patients to identify and clarify what they really want and who they want to be (White 1999). In valuing her personal autonomy, Phyllis should ask herself 'can I take responsibility for not disclosing the test result while retaining my self-respect?' In former times, Phyllis had shown a great responsibility toward her family; she was the one who took care of her mother and sister. It is because of the disappointments she has suffered that she does not feel the same responsibilities anymore. Still, Phyllis could ask herself if she really wants to stay sad and isolated.

In a relational ethic, self-determination and responsibility to others can coexist. People may exercise individual agency through their responsibility to others as Jane already seems to do. Jane says 'Once I reached my thirties and had my own two daughters things started to feel different. I worried more about developing cancer and not being there for my girls.' Jane's self is shown as a self that is connected and engaged with others.

On the other hand, questions can also be raised concerning Jane's ability to make an autonomous decision. Genetic information can strongly influence one's life and can thwart a person's autonomy. Some can become over-concerned. For instance, is Jane really as vulnerable as she claims to be? Are her worries rational or are they mistaken? Or is there a real danger that Jane is a victim of the geneticisation of society? A woman's ability to make an autonomous decision is determined not only by the amount of information offered but also by the manner in which it is communicated to her. Again, a less non-directive form of genetic counselling seems to be required. As Donchin correctly states:

In the interest of promoting women's autonomy capacities, the nondirective paradigm should give way to a nonhierarchically structured model of genetic counselling that fosters a collaborative relationship and enhances a client's capacities to exercise agency with her own relational context. (Donchin 2000: 252)

Practices of responsibility

Being responsible for someone has to do with protecting the other who is vulnerable. Goodin has defined his principle of individual responsibilities as 'if A's interests are vulnerable to B's actions and choices, B has a special responsibility to protect A's interests.' It is for this reason that parents have special responsibilities toward their children. The same could be said of the responsibilities teachers have toward their students, or doctors toward their patients.

This principle of responsibility also makes it clear why we are not always responsible at all times for everyone. We are only responsible for those who are vulnerable to our actions but the principle of responsibility is only intelligible against a background of existing practices and normative expectations. It is because of the normative expectations that we have of family life, for example, that we think that parents are responsible for their children. The assigning and accepting of responsibilities takes place within the context of a practice of responsibility in which normative expectations play an essential role. Every practice of responsibility therefore has its own geography, as Walker would put it. In a geography of responsibility we can read how and upon whom responsibilities fall and the flow of shared understandings about who is going to be expected to be accountable for situations, outcomes or tasks. In the case of family responsibilities we see expectations that we associate with family roles and we are particularly vulnerable to deep disappointment and even damage if those expectations are simply shrugged off. These expectations themselves are often based on deeply held beliefs about the cultural and moral meaning of family life and the responsibilities connected with these. Within a practice of responsibility (family, healthcare, education and so on) we make each other accountable to certain people for certain states of affairs, we define the scope and limits of our agency, affirm who in particular we are, show what we care about, and reveal who has the standing to judge and blame us. In the ways we assign, accept or deflect responsibilities we express our understandings of our own and others' identities, relationships and values.

These practices of responsibility can be analysed as gendered or infused by other power relations. A normative reflection on these practices therefore asks to investigate whether the understandings on which these practices stand can be shared by everyone involved.

It is interesting to note that the practice of genetic predictive diagnostics itself can be seen as a practice containing a certain geography of responsibility. The development in genetics and the opportunities created for healthcare alters the assignment and acceptance of responsibility. For instance, the geneticist takes this line of reasoning, when she considers genetic tests as something that belongs to the whole family: 'I feel that in these situations, Phyllis's test result really belongs to her whole family, not just to her. She has the information that is highly relevant to Jane, yet she is withholding it.' The geneticist thinks that one can only have a test on the condition that it will be all right to use the test result for the benefit of other family members.

As we have already seen, the understanding of family responsibilities is certainly not shared by Phyllis although she would probably feel and decide differently if she still felt as a member of the family. As things are now, Phyllis does not feel any family responsibility because she is estranged from the family to which she used to belong. The simple fact of Jane being family is not sufficient reason for Phyllis to disclose the genetic information. On the other hand, Phyllis seems to disregard the harm that a family member in a position of power can exert over vulnerable others. She also does not reckon with the change in assigning responsibilities as a result of new developments in genetic diagnostics.

Conclusion

I have not come up with clear answers to the issues that the case of Jane and Phyllis has raised. The care-ethics approach requires us to examine a wealth of detail about our roles, obligations and emotional commitments. What may appear to an outsider to be the morally commendable action (i.e. Phyllis's refusal to disclose genetic information to Jane), this may be viewed quite differently by the person involved who appreciates the nuances of relationships. This is in line with the concreteness that feminist care ethicists applaud in adequate moral reasoning. The most important conclusion of this chapter is that an ethical approach to genetic counselling calls for a broader sensitivity. It includes sensitivity to family dynamics, attention to the effects of social arrangements on moral understandings and experiences, and respect for agency as lived. The moral duty to disclose genetic information is something that cannot be assigned abstractly.

NOTES

1   Gilligan developed her model of moral reasoning to counter the moral development theory of Lawrence Kohlberg. The latter defined the mature moral stage as the stage in which the moral subject follows self-legislated, self-imposed and universal principles of justice (see Kohlberg 1981).
2   Care ethics can be seen as one of the candidates of an ethics of medicine and family as Hilde and James Lindemann Nelson propose (see Lindemann Nelson and Lindemann Nelson 1995).

REFERENCES

Benson, P. (2000). Feeling crazy: self-worth and the social character of responsibility: In Mackenzie and Stoljar (2000), 72–93 (see below).

Carse, A. I. and Lindemann Nelson, H. (1996). Rehabilitating care. *Kennedy Inst Ethics J*, **6**(1), 19–35.

Code, L. (1991). *What Can She Know? Feminist Theory and the Construction of Knowledge*. New York: Cornell University Press.

Dillon, R. (1992). Respect and care: toward moral integration. *Can J Philosophy*, **22**, 105–32.

Donchin, A. (2000). Autonomy and interdependence: quandaries in genetic decision making. In Mackenzie and Stoljar (2000), 239–40 (see below).

Gilligan, C. (1993). *In a Different Voice: Psychological Theory and Women's Development*. Cambridge, Mass.: Harvard University Press.

Govier, T. (1993). Self-trust, autonomy and self-esteem. *Hypatia*, **8**(1), 99–120.

Hampton, J. (1997). The wisdom of the egoist: the moral and political implications of valuing the self. *Soc Philosophy Policy*, **14**(1), 21–51.

Held, V. (1993). *Feminist Morality: Transforming Culture, Society and Politics*. Chicago: University of Chicago Press.

Hoagland, S. L. (1990). Some concerns about Nel Noddings' caring. *Hypatia*, **5**(March), 107–14.

Jaggar, A. (1989). Feminist ethics: some issues for the nineties. *J Soc Philosophy*, **20**, 91–107.

(1995). Caring as a feminist practice of moral reason. In V. Held, ed., *Justice and Care: Essential Readings in Feminist Ethics*. Boulder: Westview Press, 179–202.

Kohlberg, L. (1981). *The Philosophy of Moral Development: Moral Stages and the Idea of Justice*. San Francisco: Harper & Row.

Lindemann Nelson, H. and Lindemann Nelson, J. (1995). *The Patient in the Family*. London: Routledge.

Little, M. O. (1998). Care: from theory to orientation and back. *J Med Philosophy*, **23**(2), 90–209.

Mackenzie, C. and Stoljar, N., eds. (2000). *Relational Autonomy: Feminist Perspectives on Autonomy, Agency and the Social Self*. New York: Oxford University Press.

McCullough, L. B. (1998). Molecular medicine, managed care and the moral responsibilities of patients and physicians. *J Med Philosophy*, **23**(1), 3–9.

Meyers, D. (1989). *Self, Society and Personal Choice*. New York: Columbia University Press.

Noddings, N. (1984). *Caring: A Feminine Approach to Ethics and Moral Education*. Berkeley: University of California Press.

Reich, W. T. (1995). History of the notion of care. In W. T. Reich, ed., *Encyclopedia of Bioethics*. New York: Macmillan USA, 319–44.

Rich, A. (1980). Compulsory heterosexuality and lesbian existence. *Signs*, **5**, 631–60.

Ricoeur, P. (1992). *Oneself as Another*. Chicago: University of Chicago Press, 191.

Silvers, A. (1995). Reconciling equality to difference: caring (f)or justice for people with disabilities. *Hypatia*, **10**(1), 30–46.

Tong, R. (1996). Feminist approaches to bioethics. In S. M. Wolf, ed., *Feminism and Bioethics: Beyond Reproduction*. New York: Oxford University Press, 67–95.

Tronto, J. (1993). *Moral Boundaries: A Political Argument for an Ethics of Care*. New York: Routledge, 103.

Veatch, R. (1998). The place of care in ethical theory. *J Med Philosophy*, **23**(2), 210–24.

Walker, M. U. (1991a). Moral understandings: alternative 'epistemology' for a feminist ethics. *Hypatia*, **4**(2), 16–28.

(1991b). Partial consideration. *Ethics*, **101**(4), 758–74.

White, M. T. (1999). Making responsible decisions: an interpretive ethic for genetic decision-making. *Hastings Center Report*, **99**, 1.

Wolf, S. M., ed., (1996). *Feminism and Bioethics: Beyond Reproduction*. New York: Oxford University Press.

10

A conversational approach to the ethics of genetic testing

Michael Parker

Recognition and respect for personhood

In his book *Humanity: A Moral History of the Twentieth Century*, Jonathan Glover suggests that the inhumane treatment of human beings is made possible by the failure or refusal to see them as *persons* (Glover 2001). It does not follow from this that the ability to see people *as* persons will necessarily lead one to respect their personhood.[1] Nevertheless, it does suggest that the ability (or willingness) to recognise personhood in others, to see them as persons like ourselves, can have an important role to play in creating sensitivity to the morally relevant features of situations such as the one described by Anneke Lucassen, and it may mean that we are more likely as a result to be respectful of the personhood of those with whom we come into contact in our personal or professional lives. The demand for reciprocal recognition of and respect for personhood – that is the requirement that those making moral judgements 'place themselves in the shoes' of those about whom or for whom a decision is being made – has a long history in moral philosophy, as has another related requirement, that we should 'treat others as we would wish ourselves to be treated', the so-called Golden Rule. Why is this and why is it that the desires, wishes and interests of people are of special moral importance? To ask this question is not to call for an account of what it is that is valuable about the wishes of any *particular* person, say Jane's wishes, or those of Phyllis, but is rather to ask what it is that is especially valuable about human wishes, desires and interests per se.

One good reason for believing that special value ought to be placed on the lives of human beings is that they are *themselves* capable of valuing their lives and existence (Harris 1985: 8). What gives such lives special value on this account are the actual wishes, desires, hopes and projects of such persons.[2] It is the things that people are themselves capable of wishing to do with their

Case Analysis in Clinical Ethics, ed. Richard Ashcroft, Anneke Lucassen, Michael Parker, Marian Verkerk, Guy Widdershoven. Published by Cambridge University Press.
© Cambridge University Press 2005.

lives that make them of special moral significance (Harris 1985: 8). That people are capable of having such wishes is captured beautifully by Isaiah Berlin's famous account of 'positive liberty':

> I wish my life and my decisions to depend on myself, not on external forces of whatever kind. I wish to be the instrument of my own, not of other men's acts of will. I wish to be a subject, not an object; to be moved by reasons, by conscious purposes, which are my own, not by causes which affect me, as it were from outside. I wish to be somebody, not nobody; a doer – deciding, not being decided for, self-directed and not acted upon by external nature or by other men as if I were a thing, or an animal, or a slave incapable of playing a human role, that is of conceiving goals and policies of my own and realising them. This is at least part of what I mean when I say that I am rational, and that it is my reason that distinguishes me as a human being from the rest of the world. I wish, above all, to be conscious of myself as a thinking, willing, active being bearing responsibility for my choices and able to explain them by references to my own ideas and purposes. (Berlin 1969)

If wishes, projects, desires and hopes such as these do not provide convincing reasons for placing special moral value on a person's life, it is difficult to imagine what might.

Having a 'sense of self'

These arguments should not of course be taken as implying that only those capable of expressing themselves as eloquently as Isaiah Berlin are of moral significance. Very few, if any, of us would meet this criterion. The relevant claim here is simply that we have special reason to value those capable of valuing their own lives and this is applicable to *any* being capable of so doing. For a being to have the required sense of the future and a desire to experience that future, that is, for them to be a *person*, they do not have to be able to articulate that desire in any very sophisticated way.[3] The requirement is simply that they place some such value on their life. The way in which they do so will inevitably come in a variety of different and more or less easily recognisable forms, from the very sophisticated and well-formulated plans of Isaiah Berlin to my own very much less well-expressed plans or those of a three-year-old child.[4]

If it is accepted that beings capable of valuing their own lives should be accorded special moral respect, an obvious supplementary question arises: how might we recognise such beings when we encounter them? Following John Harris, it seems reasonable to argue that a necessary feature of any such being will be that it is in fact *aware*, to at least some degree, that it has a life to value (Harris 1985: 8) and this in turn implies that such a being would have to have a sense of personal identity, that is a 'sense of self'.

The sense of self required for personal identity is sometimes characterised as a sense of 'location' from which a person perceives the world and from which they act. Rom Harré argues that the requisite sense of location comprises three aspects – he calls these Self 1, Self 2 and Self 3 – each of which is a necessary and complementary feature of personal identity (Harré 1998: 3–4). Harré's first two aspects of self – Self 1 and Self 2 – are most immediately relevant to the preceding argument. Following Locke and Strawson he argues that in order to have a sense of personal identity, a person must have a sense of themselves as 'occupying one and only one standpoint from which to perceive and act upon the environment both external and internal' (Strawson 1969, Locke 1984, Harré 1998: 177). That is, the person needs to have a sense of him- or herself as unique, as located in space and as having a sense of 'permanence', of location in time. Harré calls this Self 1. In addition, a sense of self must also include, Harré suggests, a sense of oneself in relation to one's attributes, desires, aims and projects (Harré and Gillett 1994). Harré calls this Self 2. For Harré, this second sense of self will inevitably take a narrative or conversational form and he argues that these narratives will encompass:

. . . what sort of person one is, what one's strengths and vulnerabilities are and what one's life history has been. The concept is manifested in the self-concept which is none other than the stories one tells about oneself and the actions one performs as oneself. (Harré 1998: 177)

Self 1 and Self 2, as articulated by Harré, together describe the features of a being meeting Harris's criterion for deserving special moral respect. They describe a being with a sense of itself and of its life both as unique and as identified with a set of valued projects, aims and desires. In his account of the necessary conditions for personhood, Harris also gives central importance to self-awareness of these two kinds:

In order to value its own life a being would have to be *aware* that it has a life to value. This would at the very least require something like Locke's conception of *self-consciousness*, which involves a person's being able to 'consider itself as itself in different times and places'. Self-consciousness is not simple awareness, rather it is awareness of awareness. To value its own life, a being would have to be aware of itself as an independent centre of consciousness, existing over time with a future that it was capable of envisaging and wishing to experience. (Harris 1985: 18)

Harris draws this argument from Locke:

. . . we must consider what *person* stands for; which I think, is a thinking intelligent being, that has reason and reflection, and can consider itself, the same thinking being, in different times and places; which it does only by that consciousness which is inseparable from thinking and seems to me essential to it; it being impossible for anyone to perceive without perceiving that he does perceive. (Locke 1984)

The third necessary aspect of 'sense of self' (Self 3)

What Harré's account of Self 1 and Self 2 does not yet provide is an explanation of how such senses of self might *arise*, of what it is that makes it possible for us to come to have a 'sense of self' and of personal identity. This is relevant to the preceding discussion because an investigation of the necessary conditions for Self 1 and Self 2 reveals the necessity of a third complementary sense of self (Self 3) for the ascription of personal identity.

There is the potential for the appearance of circularity in the account set out thus far. It may appear that what Harré (and hence Harris) is claiming is that the necessary condition for awareness of self is itself self-awareness. Following George Mead and Lev Vygotsky, Harré escapes this circle by arguing that the self-awareness required for Self 1 and Self 2 is made possible by a particular kind of social interaction, the possibility of which is not in itself dependent upon self-consciousness.[5] Self-awareness, on this account, emerges from, and is hence dependent upon, the existence of certain types of social interactions. George Mead expresses this idea as follows:

The social act is a precondition of [consciousness]. The mechanisms of the social act can be traced out without introducing into it the conception of consciousness as a separate element in that act: hence the social act, in its more elementary stages or forms, is possible without, or apart from, some form of consciousness. (Mead 1974: 18)

The self, as that which can be an object to itself, is essentially a social structure, and it arises in social experience. After a self has arisen, it in a sense provides for itself its social experiences, and so we can conceive of an absolutely solitary self. But it is impossible to conceive of a self arising outside of social experience. (Mead 1974: 140)

Similarly, for Vygotsky:

The social dimension of consciousness is primary in time and in fact. The individual dimension of consciousness is derivative and secondary. (Vygotsky 1979)

Every function in the child's cultural development appears twice: first, on the social level, and later, on the individual level; first *between* people (interpsychological), and then *inside* the child (intrapsychological). This applies equally to voluntary attention, to logical memory, and to the formation of concepts. All the higher functions originate as actual relations between individual human individuals. (Vygotsky 1978: 57)

Both Vygotsky and Mead argue that the development of our sense of self is mediated by our social interactions. For them, it is only because we are *treated as if we were persons* by others that we come to *be* persons:

From the very first days of the child's development, his activities acquire a meaning of their own in a system of social behaviour and, being directed towards a definite purpose, are frequently refracted through the prism of the child's environment. The path from object to child and from child to object passes through another person. (Vygotsky 1978: 30)

We are aware of ourselves, for we are aware of others, and in the same way as we know others; and this is as it is because we in relation to ourselves are in the same [position] as others are to us. (Vygotsky 1979)

The essence of [the general law governing the development of behaviour] is that in the process of development the child begins to practice with respect to himself the same forms of behaviour that others formerly practised with respect to him. (Vygotsky 1991)

The relevance of these arguments to this chapter is that they suggest that in addition to the senses of self identified by Harris as criteria for the ascription of personhood, and described by Harré as Self 1 and Self 2, a third complementary aspect of self is required. This is a sense of self as a certain kind of *social* location. Harré calls this Self 3 (1998: 177). In addition to having a sense of location in space and time, and in relation to its desires, attributes, aims and projects, a being of this kind must have a sense of location in relation to others, that is, it must be socially located.

It is important to reiterate that it is not simply a contingent fact that our sense of self arises in a social context (Parker 2001). A sense of self is only *possible* within the context of such interactions. The necessity of this third aspect of self has important implications for the understanding of personhood, and consequently for what might be meant by 'respect for personhood'. It implies too that even those aspects of ourselves and of our 'sense of self' that we tend to think of as the most personal, private and individual have their origins in social relationships of one kind or another. This begins to undermine the credibility of the common (mis)conception of the relationship between the self and the other, in terms of a relationship between fundamentally discrete individuals, a misconception not uncommon in bioethics. This is not to suggest that there can be no such thing as an 'autonomous self' in the everyday sense of the term but it does imply that all such selves do, necessarily, have their *origins* in social interactions of particular kinds and that the *development* and flourishing of such selves is unavoidably social. We make sense of our selves and develop our sense of personal identity (and a sense of the personal identity of others) in the course of our relationships with those around us. On this revised account of selfhood (and hence of autonomy), the self does not pre-exist society or our relations with others but emerges from them and continues to be elaborated and sustained intersubjectively, throughout life. Charles Taylor expresses this idea as follows:

My self-definition is understood as an answer to the question [of] who I am. And this question finds its original sense in the interchange of speakers. I define who I am by defining where I speak from, in the family tree, in social space, in the geography of social statuses and functions, in my intimate relations to the ones I love, and also crucially in the space of moral and spiritual orientation within which my most important defining relations are lived out.

This obviously cannot be a contingent matter. There is no way we could be inducted into personhood except by being initiated into a language. We first learn our languages of moral and spiritual discernment by being initiated into an ongoing conversation by those who bring us up. The meanings that the key words first had for me are the meanings they have for *us*, that is, for me and my conversation partners together. Here a crucial feature of conversation is relevant, that in talking about something you and I make it an object for us together, that is, not just an object for me which happens also to be one for you … The object is for us in a strong sense … with the notion of a 'public' or 'common space'.

This is the sense in which one cannot be a self on one's own. I am a self only in relation to certain interlocutors: in one way in relation to the conversation partners who were essential to my achieving self-definition; in another in relation to those who are now crucial to my continuing grasp of languages of self-understanding – and, of course, these classes may overlap. A self exists only within what I call 'webs of interlocution'. (Taylor 1989)

I have suggested that this interpersonal model of personhood will have implications for what is to count as respect for persons and hence for the interpretation of the moral dimensions of cases such as that of Phyllis and Jane. In what follows I suggest that these implications fall into two over-lapping categories. First, there are implications for what are to count as respectful relationships between persons (I shall refer to this as *informal conversational ethics*). Second, and relatedly, there are, I suggest, implications for the nature of ethical decision-making processes (I shall refer to this as *formal deliberative ethics*).

Informal conversational ethics

I have argued that special moral significance ought to be given to beings capable of valuing their own lives and existence, that is, to *persons*. Following Glover, I have suggested that a moral world is one in which such beings are recognised and respected *as persons* both by themselves and by others. But what might it mean in practice to recognise and respect people as persons in the required sense in the light of the preceding discussion of personhood? One way of responding to this question might be to say that respecting persons requires us in our relationships with them, to act towards them in ways conducive to their (and our own) flourishing as persons. But what might this mean in practice?

I have suggested in this chapter that to be a person is, at least in part, to be engaged in an ongoing process of 'making sense' of one's place, or location, in the world and of one's relationships with others. Following Harré, and to some extent Mead, Taylor and Vygotsky, I have argued that this process of making sense is necessarily an intersubjective and conversational project possible only within the context of certain types of relationships with others (and with ourselves) – what Taylor calls 'webs of interlocution'. This implies that the elaboration of personhood is itself in large measure a moral quest, because on this account, at the heart of our developing sense of personal identity is an attempt to work out ways of living with those who together constitute our social location – our family, friends, colleagues, enemies, strangers and so on. My central claim is that conversation is the developmental fundamental of human moral experience and hence of personhood (Parker 1995). But not just any conversation will do and what these arguments imply is that respect for personhood (both in oneself and in others) is made possible by and embodied in our engagement in conversations with certain characteristics. These are conversations conducive to the achievement of a flourishing sense of personhood in ourselves and in others. Such conversations will be characterised by:

- an implicit or explicit orientation towards achieving respectful ways of living together. One element of this will be an implicit or explicit orientation towards the achievement of shared understanding (even if this is the agreement to disagree);
- respect for the desires and wishes of others (and ourselves);
- concern for the well-being of others (and ourselves);
- mutual engagement and interest;
- honesty and authenticity;
- fairness;
- both listening and speaking, and by the giving of and listening to reasons;
- forthrightness and willingness to disagree openly.

I have deliberately not expressed these characteristics in terms of professional–patient relationships. I shall say more about the specific implications for the doctor–patient relationship in what follows. One advantage of beginning with an account of the moral relations between persons (rather than between professionals) is that it makes it possible to provide an analysis of the personal relationships of the participants in the case, in addition to carrying out a complementary analysis of the professional context. The approach I describe is not simply a professional ethics but also a broader account of what it is to engage in relationships that both recognise and respect persons.

Formal deliberative ethics

One of the clearest implications of a commitment to respect for persons is that wherever possible decisions ought to be made by those who are going to be affected by them. I have described some of the characteristics of a process of this kind in the previous section. A practical problem faced by this approach and by all patient-centred approaches to ethics is that it is not always possible for decisions to be made by patients themselves in the context of a case-by-case conversation such as that described above. This may be for a number of reasons. It may be that the patient in a particular case is incompetent. It may be that the required decision is a systemic or policy decision, such as a decision about the appropriate allocation of resources between primary care and public health. Or it might be that a decision needs to be made in a situation in which there is a serious and intractable disagreement about fundamental values or a conflict between parties that makes conversation impossible. What are the implications of the approach sketched out in this chapter for situations in which it is not possible to base decision-making on the wishes of individual patients, for example in the setting of policy? Such situations call for the development of more formal deliberative decision-making processes. Formal deliberative processes of this kind might be expected to be both consistent with the principles of respect for persons discussed in this chapter and hence to have the following characteristics:

- The orientation of the decision-making process should be towards the establishment of a model of practice conducive to respect for and recognition of persons. In addition to placing constraints on the nature of the decision-making process, this requirement will also act as a constraint on the legitimacy of the outcomes of such a process.
- Any such process should, as far as is possible, be participatory, including those who will be affected by or have a legitimate interest in the outcome of the decision.
- The deliberations through which decisions are reached should themselves be governed by the conversational principles described in the preceding section, i.e. the principles of informal conversational ethics.
- Decision-making should focus on the exploration and consideration of reasons and the use of argument. This does not imply a separation of reason and emotion; emotions can provide good reasons.
- Fairness.
- Where it is not possible for patients to be involved in decision-making, decisions should be made according to a process that patients might be expected to accept as reasonable.
- Finally, it is an implication of the preceding arguments, that decision-making processes should be transparent and accountable (Daniels 2000). Those who make decisions should be willing to explain the decision-making process and to defend the decision made in front of those who are to be affected and should also be willing to learn from and develop the process in the light of the responses and criticisms they receive.

Implications for the case of Jane and Phyllis

I have argued in the previous two sections that respect for and recognition of persons is characterised by a willingness to engage in certain types of conversations with them and, where such conversations are not possible, by the adoption of certain types of deliberative decision-making processes. In what follows I attempt to explore the meaning of respect for persons, as defined in this way, in the case described by Anneke Lucassen.

Formal deliberative ethics

I begin with a consideration of the formal aspects of the case because it seems to me that one reason why the case is so problematic is because of the lack of prior agreement about what is to constitute good practice in situations like this, and a consequent failure on the part of the various healthcare professionals to establish with Phyllis and Jane in advance what the ground rules were to be in the clinical genetics consultation and subsequent relationships. That is, the health professionals appear to have failed to make clear to Phyllis and Jane what they could reasonably expect. Respect for persons does not always mean giving people exactly what they want but it ought to mean at the very least that Phyllis, say, should have been given a sense of the rules governing genetics practice and the reasons for them early on in the clinical encounter. My first practical conclusion, therefore, is that genetics centres, and perhaps the health service more widely, should develop policies and models of good practice setting out for health professionals, patients and their families, the principles that inform their practice. And they should be willing to defend and, if appropriate, change such principles. These should include agreements about how patients are to be informed about genetics, when tests should and should not be carried out and the rules governing the sharing (or not sharing) of genetic information with other family members (including rules about exceptions, e.g. in cases of serious harm).

Following my earlier arguments, such principles and models of good practice should themselves be developed in ways that are inclusive, accountable and reasonable. This does not necessarily mean *more,* or even very much more directive or detailed, guidelines but it does mean that health professionals have an obligation to reach some degree of broad agreement before providing a clinical service, on the principles by which that service is to be guided, and to make such principles clear to those using the service. Such principles should be reviewed regularly and there should be scope for professional judgement in the light of special morally significant features of individual cases. In addition to being developed in ways that are inclusive and reasonable, the implications of the policy must, of course, themselves be consistent with respect for persons.

One additional reason for developing models of good practice is that while some difficult situations involving conflict and uncertainty, such as, for example, the one involving Phyllis and Jane, might be avoided by discussion early on in the counselling process about, for example, how familial information is to be shared (or not shared) following a test, others will not be. The development of a general policy for such cases is important because in many cases agreement among the participants will not be possible *de novo* and also because in others, even where such agreement has been reached, people will subsequently change their minds. In such cases it is much better and more respectful if those involved know upfront what is going to happen and why, even if they disagree with it. At least the cards are on the table. In the case described by Anneke Lucassen, new cards were produced after the game had started and it is hardly surprising that Phyllis in particular feels that she has been cheated. For this reason, it is important for counsellors to clarify, before testing, what the clinic will do in situations like this, so that patients know what to expect.

So my first response to the case as presented is to say that the health professionals need to learn from this experience and develop coherent and acceptable models of good practice for the future. These should be developed in something like the ways described in the previous section and should be conveyed to patients early on in the counselling process in ways that are understandable to them.

On the specific point of whether mutational analyses should be shared, my personal view (subject to a broader debate about this deciding differently) is that the results of mutational analysis should be available for use by health professionals in the clinical care of all family members and that this should be made clear in advance to those who take tests of this kind, e.g. breast cancer (Parker and Lucassen 2004). This is not to say that information about the *illnesses, treatment or identity* of family members should be shared with other family members but that the mutation details should be available for use by clinicians where this has the potential to avoid significant harm.

I have been speaking of hypothetical future cases and future policies, but what should be done in the case of Phyllis and Jane, accepting that in an ideal world we would not be in this position? It would be too easy to avoid dealing with the case as it stands and to call for 'more discussion' or the development of a policy. But what would it be reasonable to do in this case as it stands? One broad implication of the approach I have outlined in this chapter is that a very high value should be placed on the attempt to encourage communication within families and that patients such as Jane and Phyllis should be encouraged to communicate with one another. Clinical genetics teams tend to be very experienced at working with families in this way and will usually be successful in this. However, while the health professionals in this case do appear to have made significant efforts to get communication going they seem, unfortunately, to have reached a dead end. Accepting for the sake of argument that this is the case, what should happen? Given that the rules were not spelt out to Jane and Phyllis at the start and that there is no time to establish a policy before making a decision, what would be a reasonable and justifiable way forward? That is, a way that we would be willing and able to justify to Jane and to Phyllis.

It is clear that most reasonable people would, in general, expect the health service to maintain very high standards of confidentiality and only to breach such confidentiality under extreme circumstances – one might reasonably expect both Jane and Phyllis to agree to this. This raises the question of what kind of circumstances these might be. One obvious exception to the rule of confidentiality that we might expect reasonable people to agree to, even if they place very high value on confidentiality, is where there is a chance of avoiding very serious harm or even death. One might reasonably expect both Jane and Phyllis to agree about this too. It is not clear in the case as described, for example, that Phyllis is saying that she would not want doctors to save Jane's life if they had the chance, nor that she would not wish them to save Jane from very serious disfigurement. Phyllis appears to be making a general and rather abstract statement about her willingness or unwillingness to communicate or 'have anything to do with' Jane and appears not to have been confronted with the fact that her unwillingness to share the information might lead to death or serious disfigurement of the kind confronting Jane. Perhaps in her anger or perhaps because she has not been fully informed about it, Phyllis has not really thought about this. My view is that she should have been challenged to think about this. And, were they to consider this a possibility, I would urge the doctors to arrange another meeting with Phyllis to explore this point with her further.

My reading of the case as described is that the doctors would not feel comfortable about going back to Phyllis. However, my own view is that a prophylactic mastectomy does constitute a serious disfigurement and a fifty per cent chance of avoiding it is a good reason for breaching confidentiality. In the light of this, and of my argument about what a reasonable person would expect in this situation, my preferred solution here (and recognising the need for future cases to be dealt with according to a new policy) is that, despite the difficulties, Phyllis should be contacted again and reasonable efforts made to encourage her to see the benefits of sharing information with her family members. Situations such as that facing Jane should be put to her as examples of the kinds of harm that might be avoided through the use of such information. If it continues to be clear that Phyllis is not going to allow this information to be used, she should be informed that health professionals have an obligation to breach confidentiality where there is an avoidable risk of death or serious harm and that the kinds of situations described to her would count as situations in which this would be the case, and in which information would be shared despite her wishes. It should also, of course, be made clear that what is being proposed is not the sharing of information about Phyllis's illness (or other personal details) but the use of the mutation analysis to make a presymptomatic test available. Following this, Jane should be contacted and told that the genetics team have found that they do in fact have information that makes it possible for them to carry out the test. They should then carry out the test using the familial mutation analysis and make it clear to Jane that the mutational analysis is also available for any other family member who wishes to come for presymptomatic testing.

Having dealt with this case, the team, and indeed geneticists nationally, should work with some urgency towards establishing clear rules and models of good practice in this area and should make these rules clear to patients when they come forward for testing. The process of developing such a policy should have the characteristics set out above. My own view, as I have said, is that confidentiality should be maintained but that the results of mutational analyses should be available for the care and treatment of all family members, but I am open to being persuaded differently by convincing reasons subjected to discussion in a process along the lines described in previous sections.

Informal conversational ethics

The doctor–patient relationship

Before proceeding to look at the personal relationship between Jane and Phyllis I would like to make a few comments about the implications of this model for the doctor–patient relationship. I have argued that one of the clearest implications of a commitment to respect for persons is that, wherever possible, decisions ought to be made by those who are going to be affected by them. The arguments discussed in this chapter suggest that this should *not* be taken to mean that the doctor–patient relationship should be characterised by what the Emanuels call the *informative* model (Emanuel and Emanuel 1992). That is, a model of clinical encounter based on the idea that the role of the health professional is simply to ensure that the patient is adequately informed and then to carry out the expressed wishes of the patient – a kind of idealised *non-directiveness*. On the contrary, the arguments set out in this chapter suggest that the doctor–patient relationship should be characterised by a genuine *engagement* between the doctor and patient in the collaborative attempt to achieve shared understanding (even if this is the agreement to disagree) – in the Emanuels' terms it should be a *deliberative* relationship. Such interactions should be characterised by respect; mutual engagement and interest; honesty and authenticity; compassion and sensitivity; fairness; listening and speaking on both parts; by the giving of reasons; and by forthrightness and willingness to disagree openly. This is an approach that says that respect for persons is not a passive process or a 'passing of ships in the night'. This is not a model of the doctor–patient relationship based on the usual conception of informed consent but is a model oriented towards the patient making an informed and autonomous decision through a process of conversation with an engaged and respectful interlocutor.

Patients should be encouraged to *talk through* the implications of their choices, particularly where there is the possibility of harm to others (or to themselves). Part of this will involve encouraging patients to think about the *counter-arguments* to their own position. The purpose of this is not to encourage people to change their minds but to ensure that they have really thought things through and have had an opportunity to develop their thinking on the issue at hand. This is genuinely respectful of autonomy in a way that idealised non-directiveness is not. Such an approach has implications for the way in which the relationship between the geneticist and Phyllis should have been managed and also makes it clear why the oncologist was wrong to carry out a test on Phyllis without her consent.

Personal morality

I have argued that relationships with others are crucial to our developing and sustained sense of self and personal identity and are therefore central to what is valuable and special about being a person. Nevertheless, there can be no obligation on us to enter into or to sustain an intimate relationship or conversation with another person if we do not want to do so, even if this is a close relative. If sisters do not wish to speak to one another and wish to live completely independently of one another they should be free to do so. There can be no obligation to engage in intimate relationships with people we do not like. The implication of the approach sketched out in this chapter is not that we have a duty to have relationships with particular people or even with as many people as possible. Its implication is simply that when we do enter into relationships with others we should do so in ways that are mutually respectful. Nevertheless, despite the fact that there can be no obligation to engage in relationships either in general or with specific people, it remains the case that it is in relation to others that we become persons and in relationships that our personhood develops and flourishes. What this means is that when we cut ourselves off from relationships with others, or engage in relationships that are not mutually respectful of personhood, we do ourselves harm as well as harming those others. There is a sense in which, at least at first glance, this seems to be the kind of situation in which Phyllis has ended up. In this respect, the case of Phyllis is interesting and is perhaps less clear-cut than it seems. First of all, despite the fact that she is refusing to communicate, in a sense, with the rest of her family, she has not 'cut herself off' from them. She continues to see herself and to define her sense of self in relation to them. She sees herself as a martyr, as someone who was not thanked, who was rejected and so on. She is angry with them. Despite her day-to-day isolation from her family she is in fact psychologically very deeply related to them. She punishes them by rejecting them and in rejecting them confirms her relatedness to them. She is engaged, it seems, in a kind of sadomasochistic and one-sided conversation with them. This is the very opposite of a relationship based on respect for the personhood of self and of others. This kind of 'sadomasochism' can be very pleasurable (most of us have engaged in it at one point or another) and can give an intoxicatingly strong but ultimately illusory and fragile sense of selfhood. In addition to being harmful in its own right, this is also the kind of attitude that creates the conditions for the possibility of cruelty to others and it is not coincidental that the attitude itself arises out of a perception of oneself having been disrespected.

In addition to the sense in which Phyllis's relationship with her family fails to be conducive to the flourishing of her own personhood, it is also less than ideally respectful of the personhood of others, especially Jane (although Phyllis is unaware of Jane's predicament). One of the central features of respect for persons is concern for their welfare and this implies that, other things being equal, Phyllis has an obligation to save others from risk of death or serious harm where this would come at a negligible cost to Phyllis herself.

Concluding remark

I began this chapter by arguing for the moral and social significance of the way in which we choose to see others and ourselves and of the way in which these 'ways of seeing' are embodied in communication. I have gone on to call for a particular kind of 'recognition', the mutual recognition and respect that constitute the communicative conditions under which personhood can develop and flourish. I have also, on the basis of an approach to ethics (framed in terms of respect and recognition), arrived at some practical ethical conclusions about the case of Phyllis and Jane. These conclusions in summary are:

- Geneticists and other health professionals should work towards the development of a model of good practice for dealing with the results of mutation analyses in the context of families such as the one in this case. This model of good practice should be developed in a way consistent with the constraints I have outlined above about the nature of an ethical decision-making process.
- Having developed a policy, it should be discussed with all patients who come to a genetics clinic or consider a genetic test elsewhere (e.g. oncology, neurology, paediatrics, etc.) before they consent to such a test. These conversations should conform to the principles of informal conversational ethics set out above.
- At the level of personal morality Phyllis has an obligation to save other family members (and indeed anyone else) from disfiguring surgery of the

kind requested by Jane, where to do so would come at a negligible cost to Phyllis herself.

• With respect to the case as it stands, even where no policy on the sharing of mutation analyses exists, it is reasonable to hold that there will be some situations in which it is right to breach confidentiality. In this respect I think the current guidelines are broadly correct (e.g. General Medical Council 2001). That is, where there is a risk of serious harm, breaching confidentiality (following a genuine but failed attempt to encourage Phyllis to share this information) should be allowable. Phyllis's right to define this information as confidential does not bring with it a guarantee that such information will never be shared under any circumstances. It is my view that a fifty per cent chance of a pointless mastectomy falls within the category of avoidable harm justifying a breach of confidentiality.

ACKNOWLEDGEMENTS

Thanks to Micaela Ghisleni, Anne Slowther, John McMillan, my co-editors and the contributing authors involved in this book for their comments and suggestions on earlier versions of this chapter.

NOTES

1 The fact that perception of personhood in others is by itself no guarantee of respect for such personhood is exemplified by the fact that many forms of torture and cruelty depend upon awareness of and blatant disrespect for the personhood of one person by another.

2 To suggest that persons are deserving of special moral respect should not be taken to imply that the limits of moral concern are commensurate with the relations between persons; the nature of relationships between persons is, however, the focus of this chapter.

3 In the light of Glover's study it is important not to set the hurdle for this too high as this can all to easily turn into an excuse to deny or refuse personhood.

4 This argument applies equally to any being capable of valuing its own life. It is important in this regard to take seriously Jean Piaget's insight about the differences between childhood and adult understanding. There is no necessity for childhood forms of understanding or perception of self to be the same as those of adults.

5 Axel Honneth also builds an account of interpersonal, discursive ethics on a reading of Mead. The best place to read about this is Honneth (1995).

REFERENCES

Berlin, I. (1969). Two concepts of liberty. In I. Berlin, *Four Essays on Liberty*. Oxford: Oxford University Press, 131.

Daniels, N. (2000). Accountability for reasonableness. *BMJ*, **321**, 1300–1.

Emanuel, E. J. and Emanuel, L. L. 1992. Four models of the physician–patient relationship. *JAMA*, **267**, 2221–6.

General Medical Council. (2001). *Confidentiality*. London: General Medical Council.

Glover, J. (2001). *Humanity: A Moral History of the Twentieth Century*. London: Pimlico.

Harré, R. (1998). *The Singular Self*. London: Sage.

Harré, R. and Gillett, G. (1994). *The Discursive Mind*. London: Sage 99–111.

Harris, J. (1985). *The Value of Life*. London: Routledge.

Honneth, A. (1995). *The Struggle for Recognition: The Moral Grammar of Social Conflicts*. Cambridge, Mass.: MIT Press.

Locke, J. (1984). *An Essay Concerning Human Understanding*. Glasgow: William Collins, 211. [Originally published 1690.]

Mead, G. H. (1974). *Mind, Self and Society*. Chicago: Chicago University Press. [Originally published 1934.]

Parker, M. (1995). *Growth of Understanding*. Aldershot: Avebury.

   (2001). Genetics and the interpersonal elaboration of ethics. *Theoret Med Bioethics*, **22**, 451–9.

Parker, M. and Lucassen, A. (2004). *Genetic Information: A Joint Account? BMJ*, **329**, 165–7.

Strawson, P. F. (1969). *Individuals*. London: Methuen.

Taylor, C. (1989). *Sources of the Self*. Cambridge: Cambridge University Press, 35–6.

Vygotsky, L. S. (1978). *Mind in Society*. Cambridge, Mass.: Harvard University Press.

   (1979). Consciousness as a problem of the psychology of behaviour. *Soviet Psychol*, **17**, 29.

   (1991). The genesis of the higher mental functions. In P. Light, S. Sheldon and M. Woodhead, eds., *Learning to Think*. London: Routledge, 36.

11

Families and genetic testing: the case of Jane and Phyllis from a four-principles perspective

Raanan Gillon

The four-principles approach does not purport to resolve moral dilemmas!

The four-principles approach in bioethics (beneficence, non-maleficence, respect for autonomy and justice, in case any reader does not already know them – see Beauchamp and Childress 2001 and, for example, Gillon 1994) does not purport to solve moral dilemmas resulting from conflict between the principles and thus it has no canonical response to the moral dilemma(s) presented in the case of Jane and Phyllis. While there are several obvious moral issues raised in this case, and a large variety of others that could reasonably be extracted from it, the main moral dilemma is easy enough to specify. One limb argues reasonably that the confidentiality of Phyllis's medical record should be breached in the interests of providing potential medical benefit to Jane and possibly her daughters – this horn of the dilemma pricks morally because it breaches the moral norm of medical confidentiality. The other limb of the moral dilemma argues reasonably that the strong (even though not absolute) moral norm of respecting medical confidences should be honoured and Phyllis's medical information should therefore not, without her consent, be passed on to Jane – this horn pricks morally because Jane's health, and possibly that of her daughters, may unnecessarily and possibly severely be harmed as a result of the doctors not breaching medical confidentiality.

Both limbs of this moral dilemma can be defended using a four-principles approach

Both limbs of this moral dilemma can be defended using a four-principles approach. On the one hand, preservation of medical confidentiality can be morally defended on the grounds of respect for the patient's autonomy and of

Case Analysis in Clinical Ethics, ed. Richard Ashcroft, Anneke Lucassen, Michael Parker, Marian Verkerk, Guy Widdershoven. Published by Cambridge University Press.

beneficence (and possibly too on the grounds of non-maleficence). On the other hand, by giving greater weight to beneficence over respect for autonomy and/or by increasing the estimate of benefit and reducing the estimate of harm that will be produced, the breaking of medical confidentiality will be justified, still using the four-principles approach. What then is the use of the four-principles approach it may reasonably be asked and I shall return to this question. For the time being let me simply point out that the same question can be asked of *any* approach to medical ethics that believes in the existence of moral dilemmas. And let me again at this stage simply assert that those approaches and moral theories that do not accept that there are any true moral dilemmas, which purport to be able to resolve 'apparent' moral dilemmas by an overarching method – for example, the welfare-maximising methods of utilitarianism – neither succeed in real life nor (probably) even in theory in doing so. We are stuck with the reality of moral dilemmas, and they remain moral dilemmas even after a morally acceptable method has been used to choose between the morally incompatible alternatives manifested in those dilemmas.

Given the proviso that the four-principles approach can be used to come to different moral conclusions when there are moral dilemmas (seen as describable in terms of conflicts between prima-facie moral principles and/or their derivatives) let me straight away avow my personal view as to how I would respond to the dilemma posed by the case of Phyllis and Jane, using the four-principles approach. My working life as a hybrid general practitioner and medical ethicist has sensitised me to the need to give one's own reasoned view about a problem case. Thus even if one sees justification for alternative and mutually incompatible responses, as in this case, people, especially clinicians, still generally wish to know how one would oneself respond, and one's reasons for that response, if one were having to make the decision oneself. Conversely, clinicians, who often have to make such decisions professionally, are understandably and sometimes justifiably irritated when ethicists content themselves with extensive analyses of the cases presented, explanations of their fraught and complex nature, and of the inadequacies of the way they have been handled so far.

In a nutshell, my own conclusion is that, subject to firm legal advice to the contrary, I should maintain Phyllis's medical confidentiality. However, if I were one of Phyllis's doctors, especially if I were her general practitioner, I should try hard to get her to discuss matters with me, find out more about why she does not want the test results to be passed on and then ask if she will allow me to explain why I think it could be extremely valuable for her to allow the doctors to pass the test results on. If she did allow me to have such a discussion I would explain that it is possible that her permission to reveal and use her test results could actually prevent members of her family from having unnecessary mutilating surgery. I should point out the enormous peace of mind that she could provide for any of her female relatives (who might wish to be tested and who proved not to have the familial cancer gene) and the potential benefit in terms of preventative actions that she could provide for any of her female relatives who wished to be tested and who were then found to have the familial cancer gene. I would ask Phyllis to reflect on whether she would feel at peace with herself if one of her family members subjected herself to unnecessary mutilating surgery to remove both healthy breasts and possibly both healthy ovaries to protect herself against inherited breast and/or ovarian cancer when there was a fifty-fifty chance that the need for this could be eliminated by using Phyllis's gene test. Of course I would have to be careful not to bully Phyllis – something that Alastair Campbell rightly objects to in Chapter 4 and is a major concern of Richard Ashcroft's Chapter 6. However, the use of reasoned moral argument is not in itself bullying and while I would need to be aware of, and avoid the danger of, turning a discussion between moral equals into a bullying brow-beating by a possibly personally and/or socially (as distinct from morally) more powerful doctor of a possibly weaker patient, I think it would be possible to have the discussion without bullying or brow-beating and I think it would be a discussion that I ought to ask to have.

If Phyllis asked for confidential details such as which particular family member I was concerned about, I would explain that even if I were concerned about particular family members I would be unable to talk about particular people without their permission. I would further explain that such permission would now be impossible to obtain without explaining why I wanted it, thus breaching Phyllis's own confidentiality, which I would not be prepared to do without Phyllis's own permission, just as I would not be prepared to give another family member the results of Phyllis's genetic tests without Phyllis's permission. I would earnestly entreat Phyllis to review her decision to deprive other members of her family of the use of her genetic tests if the need arose, and to trust me and other doctors to use them only in order to benefit the health of others, possibly in dramatically valuable ways either by preventing unnecessary mutilating operations or by confirming their potentially life-saving value. So I would work quite hard to influence Phyllis – by reasoned moral argument – to change her mind. (Let me add that I would also try to explore whether or not she would like to discuss the earlier problems that have led her to feel so negatively about the rest of her family: some discussions with a psychotherapist or counsellor might well prove highly beneficial to her, whether or not she gave permission for her test results to be used.) Unless and until she did change her mind and gave me permission to pass on and use her test results, I would, with enormous regret, respect her confidentiality, given the proviso about my legal obligations.

In the rest of this chapter I outline how the issue involves (among several other moral problems that I do not consider) the substantial moral dilemma as between respecting Phyllis's confidentiality at the cost of potential benefit to Jane's medical care and optimising it at the cost of breaching Phyllis's confidentiality. I look at different ways of trying to escape from the dilemma, including (very briefly) those used by other authors in this book, and I conclude that none of them (including the four-principles approach) succeeds in escaping from the dilemma. And I then outline the way I came to choose one horn of the dilemma in the decision I have just outlined.

The dilemma considered in terms of the four principles

The dilemma can be seen as representing a tension between two sets of moral arguments, each based on the four principles. On the one hand, Phyllis's confidentiality should be maintained because of the prima-facie principles of respect for autonomy (Phyllis's), beneficence (to Phyllis and to countless future patients who would benefit by respect for their privacy and thus for their medical confidences, as well as by the improved medical care that results from a strong, socially well-embedded obligation of medical confidentiality), non-maleficence (to Phyllis and to countless future patients who would be harmed by disregard for their privacy, including their medical confidences, and by the worse medical care in which failure to have a strong and socially well-embedded obligation of medical confidentiality is likely to result) and justice (to Phyllis and to all patients, who have justice-rights to privacy according to both the Universal Declaration of Human Rights (1948) and the European Convention on Human Rights, and even a probable legal right to privacy now that the latter convention is part of English law).

On the other hand, the counter-arguments that favour breaching Phyllis's confidentiality are based in beneficence (to Jane and possibly to her daughters as well as to all others who would benefit, it is here simply assumed, by having access to the genetic results of their relatives) and non-maleficence (for it is arguably maleficent of those doctors who have a duty of care to Jane and her daughters not to use their available medical knowledge to protect them from unnecessary harm, and also arguably maleficent to all future relatives of people whose genetic-test results might benefit them for their doctors to treat such results as confidential). There is also arguably an obligation in legal justice to Jane and her daughters in that their doctors have a duty of care to them that legally requires them to breach Phyllis's confidentiality to the extent necessary to protect them from unnecessary and potentially substantial harm.

Some might add that respect for Jane's autonomy also requires the doctors to breach Phyllis's confidences. However, I would argue that this belief is mistaken though it does depend on one's view of what respect for autonomy requires. A standard interpretation, which I share, is that while respect for autonomy entails a negative right that requires non-interference with the deliberated self-rule of others (in so far as such non-interference is compatible with respect for the autonomy of others) it does not entail a positive right requiring the provision of assistance to others, no matter how much they autonomously desire and request such assistance. Obligations to provide assistance to others fall under the moral principle of beneficence, including any obligations to *enhance* their autonomy. Thus, while Jane may autonomously *desire* to obtain Phyllis's medical information, respect for her autonomy does not require doctors to comply with that desire, even though it would be beneficial to Jane if they did. It is true of course that if a doctor (or anyone else) wishes to interfere with another person (for example, in order to benefit that person) then the doctor is obliged by respect for that person's autonomy to give sufficient information for the person to be able to make an adequately autonomous decision about accepting such proposed assistance, and to respect that person's decision. But it is not true, at least under this interpretation of respect for autonomy, that it requires – even prima facie – that one does what a person autonomously asks one to do.

While such cooperation is consistent with respecting that person's autonomy, and while a prior obligation of beneficence may often, prima facie, require one so to cooperate in order to benefit the person (and I have acknowledged that beneficence to Jane would require breaching Phyllis's confidences), respect for autonomy does not. It is true that some conceptions of respect for autonomy require actions to enhance others' autonomy – this is sometimes called *empowerment*. My own view is that it is both clearer and morally safer to differentiate and keep conceptually separate the duties of beneficence and respect for autonomy. Duties of empowerment are then seen as deriving from both obligations in a subset of those contexts where both obligations exist. Nonetheless even if in particular circumstances no duty of beneficence to a particular person exists or is acknowledged (and beneficence is an 'imperfect' obligation, i.e. we do not owe it to every person who could be benefited), the duty of respect for that person's autonomy remains, for it is a 'perfect' duty, i.e. owed (prima facie) to every autonomous agent.

If the duty of respect for autonomy is interpreted to *necessitate* positive obligations of beneficence, the possibility arises of denying any, even prima-facie, moral requirement to respect a person's autonomy unless one also owes that person a duty of beneficence, for if no duty of beneficence is owed to a person (and if the duty of respect for autonomy entails a component of beneficence) then no duty of respect for autonomy can be owed to that person either.

Trying to escape from the dilemma: professional and legal obligations

Given that the case of Phyllis and Jane involves this moral dilemma, this clash between mutually incompatible prima-facie moral duties owed to two people, why did I choose one limb (maintaining Phyllis's confidentiality if it was legal for me to do so and if I was unable to persuade her to give me permission to disclose her genetic-test results) rather than the other (breaching Phyllis's confidentiality in order to benefit and avoid a significant risk of unnecessary harm to Jane)? The first part of my moral analysis involved seeking (but failing) to escape from the dilemma, using a variety of reasoning processes including (briefly) those used by other contributors to this book. When faced in my medical practice with what, on preliminary analysis, appears to be a moral dilemma I tend first to assess whether or not I have any professional and/or legal obligations that at least in effect resolve the dilemma. There are two major professional and legal obligations in conflict here: a duty of care and a duty of confidentiality. Are there decisive professional and/or legal obligations that remove the dilemma by giving good moral reasons to choose one alternative rather than the other? Certainly the duty of care requires doctors to use their best efforts, including use of the best available knowledge, to optimise the treatment of their patients. However, in fulfilling their duty of care they are not required to behave either unprofessionally or unlawfully. Certainly, too, doctors are required by professional obligations stretching back to Hippocratic times to maintain medical confidences unless there are very powerful reasons to break such confidences, for example, the prevention of serious crimes such as murder and child abuse. (I have defended elsewhere the claim that the strong but prima-facie duty of medical confidentiality is easily seen to be supportable both by beneficence, individual and social, and by respect for autonomy: Gillon 1985, 1998). Would the positive benefits to Jane be sufficient to require me professionally and/or legally to breach my obligation of medical confidentiality to Phyllis? First, I reason that as it is not illegal for Phyllis to withhold her medical information from her family, even where giving such information has a fifty-per-cent chance of preventing unnecessary mutilating surgery, then:

- our social mores as represented in the law do not consider the potential harms of withholding such information as sufficient to override a general legal right to maintain one's privacy;
- it would be inconsistent for the law to allow Phyllis to maintain her privacy but it would require her doctor to override that privacy;
- that if not legally required to do so doctors, however much they disapprove of Phyllis's decision, should not go as it were above the law and in

effect override her normal legal right to maintain her privacy and to withhold her medical information from her family.

This I reason is strengthened by the fact that Phyllis will have had the medical profession's undertaking to treat medical confidentiality as a very strong obligation.

General Medical Council guidelines

How does this preliminary reasoning cohere with specific professional guidance? The General Medical Council's (GMC) guidance on confidentiality (GMC 2000) states that 'Confidentiality is central to trust between doctors and patients' and that 'Patients have a right to expect that information about them will be held in confidence by their doctors' (GMC 2000: section 1). However, it specifies various permissible exceptions to the duty of confidentiality. Obvious ones include disclosing information in order to deliver healthcare to the patient (for example, dictating a referral letter to a medical secretary). However, generally speaking, patients maintain a right to withhold their consent to disclosure and their refusal should be respected unless there are legal obligations requiring the doctor to break confidentiality or ('exceptionally') where disclosure is 'in the public interest where the benefits to an individual or to society of the disclosure outweigh the public and the patient's interest in keeping the information confidential'. This broad and imprecise criterion is made a little more precise in another section of the guidance, which explains that disclosures, despite the patient's refusal of permission, 'may be made only where they can be justified in the public interest, usually where disclosure is essential to protect the patient or someone else from risk of death or serious harm' (GMC 2000: section 4, para. 14). And the GMC adds 'Ultimately the "public interest" can be determined only by the courts; but the GMC may also require you to justify your actions if we receive a complaint about the disclosure of personal information without a patient's consent' (GMC 2000: section 4, para. 20).

Examples given by the GMC of justification for disclosure of confidential information in the public interest, despite patient refusal, are cases where patients continue to drive when medically unfit to do so and against explicit medical advice, when clinician patients place their own patients at risk because of their medical condition (for example, a serious transmissible disease or a drug addiction) or where disclosure is necessary 'for the prevention or detection of a serious crime', where serious crime is to be understood as crime that 'will put someone at risk of death or serious harm, and will usually be crimes against the person, such as abuse of children' (GMC 2000: section 5, para. 37).

Since disclosure of genetic information is not explicitly considered in the GMC guidelines or examples, were I faced with a real case such as the one we are considering, I would actually consult the GMC. However, although it seems likely that the guidance would *allow* a doctor to breach confidentiality in the case of Phyllis and Jane (for it seems clear that use of Phyllis's genetic-test results has an up to fifty-per-cent probability of preventing unnecessary and mutilating operations on Jane, and thus preventing a high risk of significant harm) I can find no reason to believe that the GMC's guidelines (at the time of writing!) would *require* any doctor to breach Phyllis's confidentiality without her consent. Rather, it seems likely that in the event of a complaint the GMC would require the doctor to demonstrate that he or she had made reasonable efforts to get consent, had considered the issues carefully, and had conscientiously judged that it was not a case where the public interest clearly *required* confidentiality to be overridden and that all in all the doctor believed that the prevention of the anticipated potential harm to another person did not 'outweigh the public and the patient's interest in keeping the information confidential' and that it was therefore a case where the norm of confidentiality should be preserved. So I conclude that the GMC advice does not in fact or in theory remove the dilemma.

British Medical Association Ethics Department guidance

In a real case of this kind I would also consult the excellent Ethics Department of the British Medical Association (BMA) and in fact I trespassed on my friendship with one of its ethics experts, Veronica English, whom I thank for the benefit of a hypothetical consultation about our hypothetical case. She drew my attention to the BMA's advice on genetics issues (BMA 1998), which reiterates that 'the doctor's duty of confidentiality to the individual patient is of fundamental importance and should only be breached when there is a legal requirement or an overriding public interest' – but it adds that in the particular context of genetic information 'individuals should be encouraged to consider the implications of their decisions for other people' (BMA 1998: 69) – and indeed in a different section the BMA advises that individuals opting for genetic testing 'should be strongly encouraged to share genetic information with those for whom it has special relevance' (BMA 1998: 71). So, for example, the oncologist who performed Phyllis's genetic test not only seems to have done so with fairly minimally informed consent to do the test at all, but also without anticipating the issue of consent to inform relatives if this became advisable: one of the many other ethical issues that this case raises and that I do not have space to discuss.

In the rare cases where permission is withheld, 'this refusal should be respected unless the limited criteria set out by the GMC are met. In such circumstances there may be grounds for breaching confidentiality' (BMA 1998: 71). The BMA book helpfully notes that the factors to be considered in coming to such a judgement will include the severity of the disorder, the level of predictability of the information provided by testing, the action (if any) available to the relatives to protect themselves or make informed reproductive decisions if they were aware of the genetic information, the levels of harm and benefit associated with giving and withholding the information, and the reasons given for refusing to share the information. If the doctor does decide to breach confidentiality he or she should, the BMA advises, at least inform the patient that such is the intention *before* doing so.

Finally, the BMA also considers the possibility that in some circumstances the doctor may have a legal *obligation* to breach confidentiality and disclose genetic information despite the patient's refusal to consent. This has not been tested in the English courts but the BMA notes that legal commentators consider it unlikely that a doctor would have a legal duty to disclose genetic information to a third party '*unless that person is also the doctor's patient*' [my italics]. In those very rare cases there might be a legal obligation (a) where the doctor has a duty of care to both patients, (b) where 'the information indicates a high probability that the relative would develop a very serious condition' and (c) where 'if the individual had the information he or she could take steps to avoid the condition or the condition could be treated'. Thus it seems clear that those doctors in the Phyllis and Jane case who had a duty of care to both of them (the GPs and arguably the geneticists, though not the oncologist) *might* even have a legal obligation to disclose Phyllis's genetic test results to Jane or at least to use them in order to test Jane. This is because (a) is fulfilled and (b) is arguably fulfilled. Of course, since Jane is intending to have prophylactic treatment even without genetic information it is not her possible breast cancer that constitutes the 'very serious condition' but it is arguable that choosing to have bilateral mastectomy with the possible addition of bilateral oophorectomy (where the operations are known to have a fifty-per-cent chance of being unnecessary) could perhaps be seen as 'developing . . . a very serious condition'. Also, (c) is fulfilled since if Jane had the information she could take steps to avoid the 'condition' (the results of the unnecessary surgery) if she proved not to have the familial breast-cancer gene herself – information that she could not obtain without her doctors first having been given Phyllis's genetic information.

Given this possibility of a legal obligation to breach Phyllis's confidentiality, my next inquiry, were I faced with the real case as Phyllis's GP or as her geneticist working in the same service as Jane's geneticist, would be to ask my medical malpractice organisation for their legal advice. In particular I would wish to have expert legal opinion about the probability that a court would find me guilty of negligence (or other legal culpability) to Jane and/or her daughters if significant harm (such as unnecessary mutilating surgery) had been suffered by any of them that could have been prevented by my disclosure of Phyllis's confidential genetic information. In this context I would ask whether bilateral mastectomy, and bilateral mastectomy plus bilateral oophorectomy would be legally regarded as in itself seriously harmful in the circumstances outlined. Although, of course, no unnecessary harm is desirable it might be arguable that even in the absence of Phyllis's confidential genetic information, overall it would still be advantageous to Jane to decide to have a prophylactic mastectomy with or without oophorectomy, and for her doctors to cooperate in providing the operation(s), although it seems clear that in the current state of knowledge none of the doctors would positively recommend the operation(s) to her even if she were found to have a specific breast-cancer gene.

To summarise, it seems likely that in the process of trying to decide, were this a real case, which horn of the moral dilemma to seize, I would be left with clear evidence that from a professional perspective I would be morally and professionally justified in either maintaining confidentiality or breaking it; while from a legal perspective, while it was not clear what a court would probably decide, a legally safer decision might be to breach Phyllis's confidentiality, since it would be very unlikely that I would be found guilty of negligence to Phyllis if I did so, given the justifications above, whereas it is possible (though uncertain) that I would be found negligent to Jane if I did not breach Phyllis's confidentiality. So, at this stage of my deliberations my preference would be to respect Phyllis's medical confidentiality if I were unable to persuade her to give me permission to use her test results. But my actual decision would depend on the legal advice given to me by my medical malpractice organisation.

Legal obligations: self-interest and morality

I have two reasons for this. The first is entirely self-interested and not particularly morally reputable, but fighting a legal case is extremely demanding of time, energy – including emotional energy – and money. If my malpractice organisation told me that I had a legal obligation to breach Phyllis's confidentiality in pursuit of my duty of care to Jane and her daughters, or that there was a sufficiently high probability that a court would so rule that the malpractice organisation would not fund my legal defence if I withheld Phyllis's genetic-test results and was then sued for negligence, then in both those circumstances I would opt to breach Phyllis's confidentiality. If, on the other hand, I was legally advised that I would have a defensible case and that my malpractice-insurance organisation would fund my legal defence if a case were brought then I would opt to maintain Phyllis's confidentiality as explained above, were I unable to persuade her to give permission for her genetic-test results to be divulged to other family members whose health might be significantly benefited.

The self-interest confessed to above is not a moral justification, merely an honest psychological evaluation of how far I would be prepared to subject myself to the burdens of a legal case in the absence of support from my defence organisation. The second and morally justified reason for my decision ultimately to depend on legal advice is that were that advice to indicate that I had a clear legal obligation to breach Phyllis's confidentiality in order to fulfil my legal duty of care to Jane (and perhaps to her daughters if they too were my patients), then that legal duty would weigh in my moral balance. Why? Because obedience to morally acceptable laws is part of the prima-facie moral obligation of justice: legal justice. Of course, the concept of a 'morally acceptable law' is both murky and contentious but it is enough to say here that provided the laws *are* morally acceptable then one has a prima-facie moral obligation to obey them. (I shall simply assert that my own admittedly unworked-out assumption is that necessary conditions for a law to be morally acceptable are that it is open to democratic revision – and thus in a sense respects the autonomy of the governed – and that it is consistent with the four universal prima-facie moral principles, but it is not a necessary condition for a law to be morally acceptable that one agrees that its substance is morally correct!)

So the law and professional ethics have not removed or dissolved the main moral dilemma presented in the case of Phyllis and Jane (whether to maintain Phyllis's medical confidences at the cost of potential serious and unnecessary harm to Jane and her daughters (and others) or to protect Jane and others from unnecessary and potentially serious harm at the cost of breaching Phyllis's confidences). Both horns of the dilemma can be defended and it seems unlikely (though possible) that either my professional or legal obligations will dissolve the dilemma or require me to seize one horn rather than the other.

Can 'scope' considerations resolve the dilemma?

Are there other ways of moral reasoning that would eliminate the moral dilemma, or at least make clear which horn to seize? Sometimes differences in the scope of application of moral obligations can function in this way. (For example, in a case of abortion a moral dilemma may be perceived in choosing between the continuing life of the fetus and the continuing health of the pregnant woman; for some of us however (but of course not all), reasoning leads us to conclude that the fetus does not have the full moral status of a person such that it does not fall within the scope of the moral obligation not to be killed unless an aggressor. If, on the other hand, we do believe that it has the full moral status accorded to persons then it does fall within the scope of that moral obligation and an abortion would not be justified unless the fetus were an aggressor against its mother and abortion were the only way of protecting her.)

In this case scope differences may well be relevant in the case of the oncologist for he has no medical duty of care to Jane (even though good practice as outlined in the BMA book would involve his encouragement to Phyllis to consider Jane and other family members) so his duty of confidentiality is not counterweighted by such a duty of care to Jane or her daughters. However, this difference in scope does not apply to the GPs or the geneticists who have a duty of care (and of confidentiality) to both Phyllis and Jane.

Still trying to eliminate or dissolve the ethical dilemma I tried a variety of other reasoning processes, including variants of most of those presented by my co-authors. My objective was to get myself out of the dilemma and into the much more morally comfortable situation where it was clear that one of the horns was morally superior to the other.

First I imagined myself in the role of the various actors in the story rather as Anneke Lucassen did in her introductory chapter. But that did not help me resolve the dilemma (except to imagine that there might be a chance of reasoning with Phyllis in a way that would result in her changing her mind about disclosure of her genetic test results to Jane and thus eliminating the dilemma). Then I asked myself if there were any good reason to give moral priority to Jane's interests rather than Phyllis's, or vice versa? (I decided that there might well have been a difference if the confidence-breaker had no special duty of confidentiality, having constructed various thought experiments in which someone who had no medical responsibilities for maintaining confidentiality could justifiably pass on information about Phyllis to Jane.) However, as argued above, the GPs and the geneticists did have duties of confidentiality and care to both Jane and Phyllis and so the dilemma remained for them. The dilemma was at least reduced for the oncologist since he had no medical duty of care to Jane to oppose his duty of confidentiality to Phyllis (though the moral dilemma remained whether simply as a well-disposed person he should break his medical obligation of confidentiality to Phyllis in order to help Jane).

Can virtue ethics resolve the dilemma?

Then I looked at the problem from a 'virtue-ethics' point of view, as Alastair Campbell does. He finds that by considering issues of trust he can resolve the dilemma in favour of maintaining confidentialty. While I come to the same conclusion, the dilemma is not resolved for me by considering issues of virtue, and in particular trust. Certainly I agree with him that it is morally desirable for patients and indeed communities to be able to rely on doctors to be trustworthy so it is of moral importance that doctors and others who have such power over lives and deaths should be worthy of that trust. But surely the dilemma remains, now re-expressed in terms of trust. The crucial question is: trust to do what? Should the doctor give moral priority to maintaining the trust of Phyllis – and by extension all patients who want to trust their doctors to maintain their confidences even if very bad consequences for others may result – or should the doctor give moral priority to maintaining the trust of Jane and by extension all patients who want to trust their doctors to use their knowledge to protect them from unnecessary and potentially dangerous surgery, even at the cost of breaking other people's confidences? Similarly, dilemmas surely remain when considering the issue in terms of other virtues such as courage, steadfastness, compassion, kindness and so on. So a virtue-ethics approach did not remove the dilemma. I acknowledge that one who firmly believed that one horn or the other of this dilemma represented the virtuous thing to do might thereby sincerely believe that the dilemma was resolved, but as I see it that reliance on a person's sincere belief is one of the weaknesses of virtue theory for sincere beliefs can often be woefully immoral. To decide what is virtuous one must have some moral criteria, for example, the four principles or utilitarianism or Kantianism or religious beliefs. Sometimes those moral criteria will conflict and this produces a moral dilemma. The dilemma can, of course, be dealt with by some sort of fiat. To call one horn more virtuous than the other is one form of fiat. My own solution is another. But mine acknowledges that the dilemma remains, that both its horns are morally justified, that it can be *virtuous* to choose either horn!

Can utilitarianism solve the dilemma?

I then looked at overall welfare, now and in the future: the utilitarian concern. Would that dissolve the moral dilemma and lead to a clear decision on the basis that breaching Phyllis's confidence produces more overall welfare and less overall harm than maintaining it? Again my answer was 'no' for I could easily see utilitarian arguments in favour of each horn of the dilemma. On the one hand, it might well maximise welfare if I broke Phyllis's confidentiality in order to save Jane from potentially life-threatening surgery that had a fifty-per-cent chance of being unnecessary. On the other hand, this sort of breach of confidentiality might further undermine trust in doctors and help undermine respect for privacy in general, and therefore reduce the overall effectiveness, and therefore benefits, of medicine in particular and overall welfare in general.

Nor am I persuaded by the general presupposition of (allegedly) morally monistic theories such as utilitarianism that there are not really such things as moral dilemmas, only apparent moral dilemmas. This utilitarian pre-supposition stems from the claims that maximisation of welfare is the overriding moral objective (rejected by many of us, even though we accept that enhancing – even in some circumstances maximising – welfare is an important moral concern) and that in any particular case there will almost always in fact be only one course of action or inaction that will maximise overall welfare. Thus according to the utilitarian perspective while we may have difficulty in finding out what that course of action or inaction is, and while this may give rise to apparent moral dilemmas, almost never will there be a real moral dilemma such that there is more than one alternative that will maximise welfare. My response to this is that even if – from God's or the Archangel's viewpoint – it were clear how to assess overall welfare, and even if it were true that in most cases of apparent moral dilemmas there were a determinate answer to the question as to which course of action would maximise overall welfare, it remains the case that we are not gods or arch-angels but mere mortals, and we are thus confronted by what seem to us to be insoluble moral dilemmas. So we have to decide how to deal with them. Should we follow a strong (for some it might even be an absolute) moral rule at the cost of some resultant major moral harm, or should we break the moral rule in the belief that this would result in more welfare? Here let me simply assert, with many others, that not only do I reject the overriding maximisation objective and the monism of utilitarianism, but also that even if I accepted both, there would recurrently arise in reality many major and minor 'apparent' moral dilemmas. These would be inevitable given our mere mortals' inability to know what course of action would maximise welfare. The dilemma would then become one of deciding when as sophisticated utilitarians we should switch from relying on our every day 'intuitive' moral thinking based on moral principles and rules (and no contemporary serious utilitarian denies the moral importance of this) into what R. M. Hare (1985) calls the level of 'critical' moral thinking based on assessment of overall welfare. In real life, especially in real medical life, these 'apparent' moral dilemmas need to be addressed, even if they are only 'apparent'. Certainly I do not find utilitarian attempts to resolve the 'apparent' moral dilemma in this case successful or convincing, for whichever horn one chooses there surely remains the 'moral residue' of having failed to do something else that it would have been good to have done; my own attempted utilitarian calculations neither eliminated this moral residue nor made it clear to me which of the two horns of the dilemma would maximise overall welfare.

Other ways of trying to resolve the dilemma

I then tried to dissolve or resolve the moral dilemma using the remaining moral perspectives presented in this book. Suffice it to assert that I did not succeed with any of them and this did not surprise me in two of the three groups of approaches that I discerned. The largest group represented in this book concentrates on understanding, presenting and explaining competing moral perspectives, whether by empirical research (empirical ethics), by exploration of people's stories (narrative ethics), by concentrating on the understandings of people's experiences (phenomenology), or on people's interpretations of their experiences and understandings (hermeneutics) or by analysing their interpersonal communications (discourse ethics). How *could* these approaches resolve or remove a genuine moral dilemma if their function is to present, explain and interpret different moral perspectives? For if those perspectives concerning a particular case are truly mutually incompatible – the nature of a genuine moral dilemma – then no amount of presenting, explaining or interpreting can make them compatible. Of course, these approaches are tremendously important in elucidating those perspectives and establishing whether or not there really are incompatibilities rather than, for example, misunderstandings. But when there are incompatibilities – including genuine moral dilemmas – then they can be removed only if one or more of the competing perspectives changes sufficiently. This, of course, is not to deny the enormous importance in moral analysis of a good understanding of the different moral perspectives in each case. It is to assert, however, that when those different perspectives do entail genuine moral dilemmas, the process or achievement of understanding those perspectives, no matter how thorough, cannot dissolve or remove the moral dilemmas, either in general or in the particular case we were given to analyse.

The second group of approaches that I identified (a group of two) was concerned, at least implicitly, with promoting the moral perspectives and interests of particular groups, either women in the case of feminist ethics or more broadly of the relatively powerless in opposition to the relatively powerful, as in 'power ethics'. In terms of the four principles such approaches can be seen as giving priority to one or other of these principles. Thus amongst the varieties of feminist ethics addressed by Marian Verkerk some – so-called 'feminine ethics' – give priority to caring within relationships (which I would identify as prioritising beneficence and non-maleficence, within a limited scope of application, over the other two of the four principles). Other feminist approaches are concerned with redressing wrongs and liberating women from male oppression. I would categorise this, though perhaps not many feminists would, as the pursuit of justice for women, in my mind an important and admirable pursuit and entirely compatible with the four-principles approach to ethics.

In so far as there is a normative claim in Chapter 6 on power ethics, it is a very tentative one; most of the paper comprises an analysis of several accounts of power relationships, and is 'better understood as preparatory to an ethical understanding of the case' and thus fits better into the first group of approaches that seek better understanding of different ethical perspectives. However, conidering that concerns about power relationships are often morally based on moral antagonism to abuse of power by those who have it, 'power ethics' when it is normative may be seen as not merely explaining but also promoting the moral perspectives and interests of the relatively disempowered. To the extent that they do so they may be seen, in four-principles terms, to prioritise the pursuit of (a particular account of) justice. But in both of these accounts I was not persuaded (and indeed neither author seemed to be persuaded either!) that the approach resolved the moral dilemma under discussion. Thus, as both Phyllis and Jane are women an approach that prioritises the interests of women is from the start unlikely to help resolve this particular dilemma; prioritising relationship perspectives, and especially those of caring relationships within families, might be argued to favour Jane's moral interests over Phyllis's. Alternatively, one of the wide-spread harms suffered by women worldwide is to have their personal interests subjugated to the interests of their families and redressing this might favour Phyllis's interests. Certainly I was unconvinced that any variant of feminist ethics could resolve the particular dilemma that we are faced with, and in Chapter 9 Marian Verkerk comes to a similar conclusion.

In so far as 'power ethics' seeks to promote the interests of the under-empowered it might be argued that Phyllis is less empowered than Jane, but Ashcroft was certainly not arguing for this conclusion and another inter-pretation might see Jane as suffering from the combined power of Phyllis and the institutional power of medical ethics. The dilemma seems unlikely to be resolved by 'power ethics'.

The third group of approaches in this book that I discerned was the group of one representing 'post-structuralist ethics'. I have a variety of concerns about 'postmodern' ethics in general (of which post-structuralist ethics is a subgroup), of which the most important is a concern about their tendency to moral relativism. However, Rob Withers' main objective (in Chapter 7) seems to be to undermine, along with Foucault and Derrida, the possibility of autonomous people existing who can autonomously control their own actions. The 'post-structuralist' understanding of people sees us/them as incomplete and vulnerable, and asserts that ethics needs to be based on an understanding of such weakness and variability. But, of course, there need be no contradiction between the existence of autonomous people and the fact that this autonomy is partial, that it is vulnerable to a wide range of assaults, and that its extent varies both within any individual at different times and in different circumstances, and between individuals. Recognising this in no way requires us, however, to ignore the moral importance of people's autonomy, nor does it help to resolve the particular moral dilemma in this case, nor moral dilemmas in general.

Let me reiterate that while I found all the other approaches in this book insightful and wise, they were unsuccessful in resolving or removing the particular moral dilemma of Jane and Phyllis, just as the four-principles approach was unsuccessful. In my view the dilemma remained and remains.

The dilemma remains: using a sort of casuistry to choose between the horns

So why did I come to the conclusion already stated, choosing to be impaled (without enthusiasm I must admit) by one horn of the dilemma rather than the other? During the interesting team discussions with editors and fellow authors of this book one sceptic suggested that I simply had a prior intuitive (or other sort of) preference for one horn of the dilemma and that I then 'fixed' the four-principles approach to support it. Let me assure the reader, as I did the sceptic, that this was not the case. I had not considered this case previously and while it did not take long to identify it as involving at least one major moral dilemma (by which I simply mean that there are good moral justifications for mutually incompatible moral conclusions) it took me a long time and much argument to and fro to decide what I think I ought to do in such circumstances. In the process of this argument (mostly with myself but also with others) I changed my mind about how to avoid this problem in future (I had previously been inclined to support the idea of making it a condition of genetic testing that other family members should have access to the results if it would benefit them) and I veered between the two horns of the present dilemma. So no, I definitely did not have a prior conclusion that I was intent on supporting. But even if I had had, it would still have been important to challenge the prior conclusion with the arguments for alternative viewpoints, and to be prepared to change the prior conclusion if the arguments against it were conclusive.

I believe that the best we can do with genuine moral dilemmas is to use some morally acceptable method for choosing one horn rather than the other. My own approach is to use a version of casuistry, which is understood as the application of general principles to particular cases in the light of clear or 'paradigm' cases. Thus the paradigm cases for this dilemma are, for confidentiality, the ordinary doctor–patient interactions in which it is mutually understood that, in general, doctors ought to preserve their patients' confidences unless there are very strong moral reasons to override confidentiality. For overriding medical confidentiality, paradigm cases include those where there is a high probability of protecting people's lives or protecting them from severe harm, or where there is a strong prima-facie obligation to respect one's (morally justified) legal obligations. Conversely, in a paradigm case of fulfilling one's medical duty of care, a doctor uses his or her available knowledge to further the medical interests of the patient. But again, paradigm cases indicate the limits of that duty of care. For example, a duty not to invade another's privacy may limit the extent to which knowledge may be pursued in order to further the medical interests of one's patient. Suppose, for example, the doctor did not have Phyllis's genetic-test result but knew that it was in a safe in her flat. Should the doctor or Jane break into the flat, break open the safe and obtain the information, on the grounds that preventing potential harm to Jane was morally clearly more important that respecting Phyllis's irrational desire for privacy? No, this would be a clear or paradigm case in which both the doctor and Jane should respect Phyllis's right to privacy, which is in such a case protected by law. But if Phyllis's right to keep her genetic information private is protected by law in that case, why should doctors be allowed to override that right? And if the agreement under which they themselves obtained the private genetic information was that it was to be used for Phyllis's medical care, with at least an implicit promise that the information would not be used for any other purpose without Phyllis's consent, doesn't the case against breaking that agreement become even stronger? To make the point more vividly, imagine a doctor gaining admission to Phyllis's flat and then to her safe on the grounds that he would use his medical skills to help her medically (perhaps she was suffering an attack of asthma and called her GP, telling him that her nebuliser was locked in the safe and giving him the combination!). Having cured her asthma should he feel entitled, even perhaps morally obliged, to take the genetic information from the safe in order to benefit Jane, despite Phyllis's refusal to grant him permission to do so? Surely not. By looking at such imaginary but clear or paradigm cases I decided that on balance I would respect Phyllis's confidentiality with the provisos I have described.

Some additional checks

But the critical reasoning was not quite over. Several checks remained. Had I, I asked myself, made my final decision on the basis of mere arbitrary preference for, or prejudice against, one patient rather than the other? No. Maybe on the basis of mere convenience or other merely self-interested consideration for the doctor? Well, I have confessed that there were self-interested limits to the extent that that I was prepared expend time, money and energy on defending myself in court if my professional defence organisation was not prepared to support my decision. While there probably is a moral defence for that degree of self-interest, my main moral justification for 'going with the law' was the important prima-facie moral obligation for us all, but perhaps especially those with powers over life and death, to do so. Then I asked myself some of the remaining questions recommended by Beauchamp and Childress in the context of trying to 'balance' competing moral claims (Beauchamp and Childress 2001: 19–20). Did Phyllis or Jane have a right that the doctor should decide in her favour (rights being particularly strong moral claims)? Well, both had prima-facie rights, one a right that the doctors should preserve her confidentiality, the other a right that the doctors should use their available knowledge to protect her from unnecessary medically inflicted harm. But this competition between their rights did not give me good reason to favour one or other horn of the dilemma. Would infringing either of the competing moral obligations have a significantly better chance of achieving the other moral goal? Again there seemed to be no substantial difference. Were there any morally preferable alternative courses of action? Yes, if Phyllis could be persuaded – without bullying and coercion – to waive her confidentiality, otherwise I cannot think of one. Were there any ways of minimising the negative effects of infringing one or other of the moral obligations? In the case of breaching Phyllis's confidentiality the negative effects would be somewhat reduced by explaining in advance what one intended to do and why, and perhaps by suggesting that she might wish to seek legal advice and by reaffirming my medical commitment to her, despite breaching her confidentiality in this case in order to fulfil my medical commitment to other patients in her family. In the case of Jane, an equivalently full explanation would probably be self-defeating by having the effect of breaching Phyllis's confidentiality. However, if one decided not to breach Phyllis's confidentiality one could help to minimise the negative effects on Jane by assessing the best evidence for and against the prophylactic operations that she is inclined to have and discussing and advising accordingly, and by regular and thorough screening, given the acknowledged family history, so that any signs of early cancer would be promptly acted upon.

So, finally, I was left with the decision to deal with the moral dilemma by maintaining Phyllis's confidentiality – in the absence of strong legal advice to the contrary and in the absence of success in trying to persuade Phyllis to change her mind – without bullying or coercing her.

A concluding reflection

I now present a final reflection about the four-principles approach in relation to the other approaches described in this book. Each of the other approaches emphasises important aspects of moral decision-making with which the four-principles approach is entirely consistent. For example, virtue theory reminds us that good people – virtuous characters – are vital to the moral life and, conversely, that the best of moral principles require good characters to enact them within a continuing and sustainable moral community. Utilitarian theories remind us of the importance of aiming for good consequences and at avoiding bad consequences and *other things being equal* of the importance of trying to maximise the good consequences and minimise the bad consequences. The moral importance of optimising our understanding of people's often complex perspectives and contexts is emphasised by approaches such as narrative ethics, discourse ethics and hermeneutics. And several of the contributions in this book have emphasised the dangers of giving excessive weight to one of the four principles, notably respect for autonomy, and particularly to a very 'thin' account of this principle that encourages an atomistic and self-centred approach to ethics in which individuals ignore the interests of others, of their communities and especially of those who are powerless, vulnerable, oppressed or maginalised. Suffice it to say that all this is entirely consistent with the four-principles approach and that I have never read an account by an advocate of the four-principles approach that offers either this travesty of an account of respect for autonomy or a claim for the overriding priority of respect for autonomy over the other three principles (such an account would describe a one-principle approach to ethics not a four-principles approach).

I have long been interested to discover any good reasons either for rejecting one or more of the four prima-facie principles, or for adding to them additional principles on the grounds that these additional principles are morally desirable and cannot be derived from one, or from some combination, of the four principles. I shall merely assert that I did not discover any such reasons or any such additional principles in the alternative approaches described in this book. As stated there was a vast amount of wisdom in those contributions – but none of it (assuming that my interpretation of the post-structuralist account as non-relativistic is correct) was inconsistent with acceptance of a four-principles account – and in so far as any of these approaches made substantive moral claims each claim could be explained in terms of one or more of the four principles.

But as I asked at the beginning, why bother with the four-principles approach if it cannot give a categorical answer in moral dilemmas such as the one in the case of Phyllis and Jane? My positive answer is that in many cases of moral analysis such dilemmas do not arise and the basic moral commitments represented by the four principles do guide us to a morally correct solution. Where dilemmas do arise I believe the four-principles approach remains helpful in enabling us to share – regardless of our cultural, philosophical, national or religious backgrounds – a set of common prima-facie moral commitments, a common moral vocabulary and a common basis for description and analysis of the moral quandary. While the approach does not purport to give us a system for resolving or dissolving genuine moral dilemmas such as the one discussed above, neither do most of the other approaches described in this book, and I have offered reasons for questioning the moral methodology of the two approaches in this book that do purport to resolve the dilemma: utilitarianism and virtue ethics (each interestingly but unsurprisingly contradicting the other as to the morally correct answer). More generally, the four-principles approach, along with pluralist approaches to ethics in general, accept that genuine moral dilemmas do exist and that there is no widely accepted method for resolving or dissolving them. I have examined my own approach to dealing with them when they arise by analysing my response to an aspect of the case of Phyllis and Jane, but I have consistently acknowledged that there is a strong moral case to be made for reaching the opposite moral conclusion from my own. It would surely be unwise, however, to reject what are widely accepted to be four basic general moral commitments because they may conflict and produce genuine moral dilemmas. Rather, I believe we bioethicists should work on development of widely and preferably mutually acceptable ways of dealing with such dilemmas when they arise.

REFERENCES

Beauchamp, T. and Childress, J. (2001). *Principles of Biomedical Ethics*, 5th edn. Oxford: Oxford University Press.

British Medical Association. (1998). *Human Genetics: Choice and Responsibility*. Oxford: Oxford University Press.

Convention for the Protection of Human Rights and Fundamental Freedoms. http:// conventions.coe.int/treaty/en/Treatises/html/005.htm

General Medical Council. (2000). *Guidance on Confidentiality*. London: GMC. (Also available on GMC website www.gmc-uk.org)

Gillon, R. (1985). *Philosophical Medical Ethics*. Chichester: Wiley, 106–12.

(1994). Medical ethics: four principles plus attention to scope. *BMJ*, **309**, 184–8.

(1998). Confidentiality. In H. Kuhse and P. Singer, eds., *A Companion to Bioethics*. Oxford: Blackwell, 425–31.

Hare, R. M. (1985). *Moral Thinking*. Oxford: Oxford University Press.

Universal Declaration of Human Rights. (1948). http://www.un.org/Overview/ rights.html

12

A phenomenological approach to bioethics

George Agich

Phenomenology is a diverse and complex philosophical movement encompassing a broad range of philosophical concerns that are linked to a common method and orientation (Spiegelberg 1982). The so-called phenomenological method involves a commitment to focus philosophical analysis and discourse on the things themselves, as they are experienced in consciousness. The phenomenological method is applicable to various specialised fields including psychological aspects of consciousness such as perception, memory, imagination or cognition, as well as everyday experience. For present purposes, I shall not discuss the complex theory of consciousness and method that divides the phenomenological movement into different branches (Spiegelberg 1982). Instead, I shall show how the phenomenological method can be useful in analysing the case of Jane and Phyllis described in Chapter 1. In order to do so, I shall discuss three related topics: the phenomenological view of experience and method; the structure of typifications or taken-for-granted background meanings that structure bioethical analysis and discourse; and elements of the case example chosen to illustrate a phenomenological approach.

Experience and method

The locus of our everyday experience is the life world of the *natural attitude* (Husserl 1967), which involves the taken-for-granted set of meanings that define the common-sense world of everyday life (Schutz and Luckman 1973). The world of the natural attitude is shaped socially.

Experience of the world and its objects is always structured by meanings that are themselves correlated (in intentionality) with acts of consciousness. All experience is permeated with meaning. The objects of everyday experience are richly laden with complex layers of meaning that are historical, personal and social in nature. For example, the object in the jeweller's window is

Case Analysis in Clinical Ethics, ed. Richard Ashcroft, Anneke Lucassen, Michael Parker, Marian Verkerk, Guy Widdershoven. Published by Cambridge University Press.

experienced not only as a gold watch of a distinctive design but as a watch that would please my wife. The watch appears not only as an object for potential purchase but also as a gift signifying either my love or a token of my request for forgiveness for some failing. These personal meanings are shaped by one's personal experiences that include one's wants, desires, choices, fears, etc. Social meanings are shaped by a shared history that brings a common-sense meaningfulness to everyday experience. This can include specialised fields of knowledge such as the history of chronography, mechanics, chemistry or physics. The gold watch, for example, has a conventional meaning in our society as both timepiece and jewellery. In our example, it further includes the subjective meanings that a unique biographical situation can bring to it. The world of the natural attitude is a taken-for-granted world whose meanings are 'on the surface'. Meanings are not isolated but function within broad contexts.

We typically assume when we see a car that it has an engine. In fact, this typification is so strong that we enter cars expecting the motor to start because cars have a degree of reliability, which encourages this expectation. When the car fails to start, we seldom assume that it lacks a motor but instead think that the battery or some other part is malfunctioning. We thus typically experience the world in terms of pre-reflective meanings. These meanings are established historically and socially (Schutz 1967, Schutz and Luckman 1973). They are sedimented in our personal and professional experience as well as in our analytical language. They incorporate and reflect cultural, ethnic and religious values and meanings, and they incorporate our unique psychosocial histories and values as well.

Experience exhibits a theme-background structure (Gurwitsch 1978). Generally, we experience the world in terms of specific objects that are the focus of our attention but these objects stand out from background meanings that provide an interpretive context or field of meaningfulness for our experience. The development of bioethics has provided such a context that has introduced specific ethical meanings into clinical medicine. This context is evident in the case presented in Chapter 2, for example, in the story of the GP and the geneticist who use bioethical concepts in their stories.

Viewing the case phenomenologically cautions us about accepting uncritically any single element as 'the' definitive problem. To do so would assume, without justification, that there is a privileged perspective. Phenomenology questions the presumption that there is or can be a privileged perspective. It helps us to avoid the temptation to see the ethics of clinical medicine as pre-given in terms of the standard problems and issues such as rights to information, informed consent or confidentiality. This caution is admittedly hard to observe because the storytellers in this case themselves allude to these 'problems' as each of the storytellers speak of tension, uncertainty and concern. Whether this underlying tension or conflict is best articulated in terms of patient rights is, of course, a question for further discussion. The phenomenological method thus places the comfortable and common modes of ethical analysis into brackets. It allows these concepts to operate under the condition that they have only provisional validity and are not allowed to shape the interpretation of the case. A phenomenological approach asks that we listen to what is latent in the stories in order to hear what is left unsaid, what is beyond, behind and implicit in what each story-teller articulates.

Structures of meaning

The case involves five stories told from different perspectives about over-lapping sets of facts and beliefs. It is not the same story told by different individuals but it is five different, though related, stories that share common themes, concerns, problems and issues. Several bioethical questions are presented in these stories. There is the question of the right of a patient to have receive full disclosure of information about the medical condition, available diagnostic testing, alternatives to that testing, as well as available treatment options and the relative benefits and risks of the treatment alternatives. Correlative to the patient's right to informed consent are duties, for example, the duty of the primary-care physician to refer the patient for genetic counselling if the clinical question is beyond the GP's professional capacity and the professional duty of confidentiality. Other questions, such as which standards of care apply and do those standards of care reflect defensible ethical values, are more deeply embedded in the case.

The clinical ethical problem presented in these stories involves Jane's concern about her propensity to develop breast cancer based on her family history. Reacting to the plethora of information that she and other women are provided with as a matter of public health education regarding prevention and treatment of breast cancer, e.g. regular breast examination and mammography, she is understandably anxious about her chances of developing a fatal cancer given her family history. The question involves Jane's chances of developing cancer, the genetic basis for that probability, which includes the family history involving her aunt, as well as her treatment options. Surrounding this thematic concern are the concerns about confidentiality of medical information, informed consent and confidentiality of genetic information. These issues are fairly standard bioethics concerns but they emerge in the case through a set of overlapping stories. Identifying these issues as bioethical involves the imposition of an interpretive framework. Some elements of this framework are *in the stories* while other elements have to be introduced into the analysis in order to engender a bioethical analysis.

A phenomenological approach to this case can help to clarify what meanings are present in the case itself and to distinguish them from those meanings that are brought into the case in an effort to analyse, clarify and resolve the conflicts or dilemmas. Such an approach can be helpful because disagreement about the ethical issues can exist at the level of the case itself or its interpretation. This case is remarkable in that the ethical questions are ready to hand, though not yet analysed or fully discussed, in the stories. A phenomenological approach to a clinical case will normally consider a number of different ways of defining themes for investigation.

Social assumptions about breast cancer are operative in the case and they influence our reading of the stories. Questions – such as 'do women have a right to information about the disease?' and 'who is responsible for providing it?' – are typically raised by bioethicists. These questions, however, will not occupy us here except to note that a phenomenological approach always attempts to identify the considerations that structure the background of the case. These considerations can, of course, be investigated or discussed in their own right. A bioethicist in approaching this case could choose to focus on the question of information about breast cancer as a matter of public health just as easily as focusing on Jane's existential dilemma.

Another example involves patients' rights. This theme emerges in the way the stories are presented. Jane's aunt, Phyllis, notably claims a set of rights. Her story questions whether the oncologist violated her right to informed consent when he apparently took a blood test without her explicit consent. By her own telling, she was not opposed to this test but it is clear that she was not fully informed of the risks and benefits associated with the testing. In this connection, the geneticist comments that this testing may have been inappropriate and he attributes it to an 'overzealous' oncologist. Phyllis's story illustrates another right, namely a privacy right regarding her own medical history and the results of diagnostic testing. She is reluctant to disclose her test result to her family who she believes, correctly or not, failed to appreciate the care she provided for her mother and sister (mother of Jane) who both died of breast cancer. The GP and partner affirm another side of the privacy right: the professional obligation of patient confidentiality. Based on it, they agree that Jane should not be informed even if it makes a difference regarding whether or not she will decide to undergo disfiguring surgery. Their attitude thus raises a question about whether confidentiality or privacy obligations can ever be overridden, which immediately refers to the historical and interpretive background of confidentiality, informed consent and privacy taking us into the realms of history and law as well as ethics.

Also at play is the well-recognised conflict in bioethics between an ethic predicated on patient autonomy and a professional ethic predicated on beneficence. Recognition of the fact that the analysis provided by the GP and partner exhibits a traditional understanding of professional medical ethics that is somewhat at odds with a patient-centred ethic of autonomy that features the language of (legal) rights is made understandable, because phenomenology shows how background beliefs, values and meanings structure our foreground interpretations and experiences. This occurs both for the protagonists in the case as well as for those of us who approach the case bringing their own background assumptions. Keeping the background assumptions, beliefs and commitments in view is an important aspect of the phenomenological method as applied to bioethical analysis and argumentation.

The difficulties associated with this case in part revolve around the important question of evidence regarding what is called a 'rogue' gene and the implication of this evidence on outcome. This is important phenomenologically. Phenomenology is centrally committed to understanding the nature of evidence. Evidence is a feature of consciousness; it includes the multitude types of experience and is not reducible to empirical data alone. Phenomenology has a well-developed theory of evidence (Husserl 1969, Zaner 1973) that makes phenomenologists sensitive to the experiences, meanings or reasons that underlie choices and beliefs. The case is structured by beliefs and attitudes about genetic disease that involve complex clinical, familial, individual and scientific understandings, and the valences associated with these factors. These understandings or interpretations of genetic disease, breast cancer and genetic testing create expectations that range from simplistic beliefs about the predictive power of genetic tests to first-hand knowledge of the devastating consequences of end-stage breast cancer and the psychological/emotional impact of breast cancer on patients and their families.

This case is thus portrayed with different voices, telling interrelated stories. It illustrates an important phenomenological feature of all clinical ethics cases, namely, that the ethics of medical practice often involve the complex and preliminary problem of delineating what constitutes the problem or matter that is, or should be, the focus of the ethical analysis. These stories thus present less an 'objective' statement of 'the' ethical problem(s) than a one-sided and incomplete portrayal of the events, actions, omissions, options, benefits and burdens of diagnostic testing, medical and surgical treatments, and counselling of patients.

A phenomenological analysis

This case begins as many bioethics cases begin with a preface characterising the issues involved. Cases that have any currency in the bioethics literature are ones that illustrate problems or issues that are generally accepted. They are understandable in terms of standard ethical concepts and principles; these cases typically are highlighted because they exemplify these categories of ethical thought that are important for bioethicists. The preface to the stories states that genetic information about one person reveals information about genetic relatives to a greater or lesser extent. Family information, we are told, raises new and profound questions about the legal and ethical obligations of health professional to disclose genetic information to at-risk relatives. We are further told 'there is conflict between preserving the confidentiality of one patient and the principle of doing no harm to another patient.' Thus, the stories that follow are pre-interpreted as a case involving a conflict of confidentiality and a principle of beneficence across generations and between family members.

This definition of problems in the preface is phenomenologically placed in brackets, that is, they are retained as a provisional characterisation of the stories that follow but will not be allowed to completely define the stories. Instead, a phenomenological approach is designed to force the bioethicist to hear the stories and make up the case *in their own terms* before imposing a bioethical interpretation. Seen in this light, we recognise that this case presentation is far removed from the actual actions, thoughts and experiences that made up the actual unfolding clinical events, assuming, of course, that these stories are anchored in actual experience. The case we are dealing with is a text in which five individuals tell their stories. We do not know how the stories were elicited or constructed. Did the problem of genetic information and confidentiality guide the selection of the stories or were the stories constructed to illustrate these particular bioethical problems? To the reader of this case and the analytical chapters comprising this book, it should be clear that the case was developed to provide a basis for illustrating alternative bioethical approaches, but within this overall project the case itself introduces specific concerns. How the stories were actually constructed is thus less important than the general point that all cases are presented in a specific way that shapes one's experiences, expectations and interpretations. Bioethical analysis is not always after the fact; its concepts can permeate and structure how a case is seen and presented in the first place. From a phenomenological perspective, the 'facts' of the case are simply those meanings that are accepted or taken for granted without question or analysis. In this sense, the facts are not immutable or objective but intersubjective. They are given meaning in and through a shared social experience. They are thus more like 'constructions' of consciousness than truly objective features of reality. The certainty that attaches to facts arises from our unquestioning acceptance of them.

Using a phenomenological approach requires that we become concerned about the evidence for our beliefs and first impressions of the case. Evidence as a phenomenological concept is not something that is in the world, but rather is a feature of consciousness. As a result, there are hierarchies of evidence. A reader of my analysis, for example, can return to the text of the case itself to see if I have 'accurately characterised it'. If I say that Jane makes a specific claim, one can return to the text to see if Jane made the claim as reported. In a similar fashion, one can ask whether Jane (assuming of course that this is a 'real' case rather than a constructed or invented one) *really* said what is reported. A phenomenologically motivated bioethicist would recognise the provisional nature of the various types of evidence that might be identified in the case.

The geneticist does not believe that testing Jane alone can provide reliable evidence, but nonetheless leans towards supporting mastectomy. What explains this posture? There is little scientific evidence to support mastectomy alone as achieving an improved outcome, so non-medical values must be at work that neither the GPs nor geneticists fully appreciate. It is generally acknowledged in bioethics that when non-medical values are used in making a medical decision, they should come from the patient rather than the physician. When they come from the physician, medical paternalism occurs because they can efface patient autonomy. It appears, then, that the GP and partner are inclined to oppose the surgery, whereas the geneticist believes that 'there is enough evidence to suggest that it is *likely* to be a benefit'. Phenomenologically, one should ask whether this statement itself is supported by evidence. When the geneticist speaks of the predictive power of genetic tests, she uses the language of probability and chance. These claims are grounded in a scientific knowledge of the expression of genes and statistical probabilities. This way of thinking underlies her belief that mastectomy is *likely* to be a benefit even though her conclusion involves non-medical values. However, because of the knowledge of Phyllis's case, the geneticist believes that for Jane there is a fifty-per-cent chance that a mastectomy is not needed. The question thus centres upon whether Phyllis's test belongs to her alone or to the family.

Our typical understandings of why medical information is confidential are at stake. The taken-for-granted answer is that information gathered in the confines of a physician–patient relationship should remain within that relationship. Unless the patient consents, medical information should not be disclosed. The geneticist, however, asks whether this traditional understanding of confidentiality is applicable in situations of genetic knowledge. Our understanding of medical confidentiality and privacy developed before the genetic revolution, which introduced a different paradigm for understanding disease. In part, the bioethical conflicts presented in this case are generated by the interplay of traditional understandings of medical ethics with genetically based diagnoses. Genetic understanding of disease and diagnosis alters the understanding of disease and raises the question about the agency of the physician dealing with genetic disease. Should the primary loyalty be with the patient or with the [potentially] affected members of the family?

In this case, the traditional principle of beneficence suggests that Jane should be advised to avoid surgery. The avoidance of the harm associated with an unnecessary surgery overrides the confidentiality owed to Phyllis. This does not mean that Phyllis's medical information can be directly disclosed to Jane but the information influencing the professional recommendation against surgery can be conveyed in general terms. If Jane insists further, the physicians can simply say that they cannot disclose the evidence for their judgement because of medical confidentiality. She should be counselled that it is not in her best interest based on all the information that the physicians possess.

This recommendation flies in the face of the standard interpretation of autonomy that sees autonomy as defined in a sphere of individual rights. On this standard view, autonomous action consists in the enactment of decisions rationally made by isolated and mature individuals. Actual autonomy, however, deviates significantly from this ideal. Actual autonomy reflects the formed identifications that define individuals as unique agents in the world (Agich 1993, 2004). These identifications involved and are based upon interactions with others. Positive interactions shape affirmative values but not all interactions bear positive valence. Phyllis reports resentment, based on what she perceived as past injustice and unfair treatment by her family. Jane's own story demonstrates that she did not have strong positive feelings about her aunt. Jane does not mention the care that Phyllis allegedly provided to Jane's mother at the end of her life. Rather than establishing grounds for differentiation, these connections demonstrate that these psychosocial relationships are complex. In their biological relationship, Jane and Phyllis share genetic information that defines who they are in a non-unique fashion. The concept of actual autonomy challenges us to think about autonomy beyond the isolated individual. The concept of actual autonomy reminds us that individuals are not completely independent but are linked by biology and family. To insist that information that is not uniquely one's own deserves full protection enlarges the sphere of confidentiality beyond the typical zone of privacy identified by some thinkers. Further analysis of this situation might suggest that an ethical choice must be made between the unique claims of individuals regarded in isolation from the claims of individuals regarded as standing in relationships. This line of analysis, however, must come to terms with the reality of the family situation in this case. Clearly, there is not a strong positive familial relationship between Jane and Phyllis. Does this fact alter the relationship based on biology?

It is worth pointing out that this case presents a fertile field for psychological interpretation that would be relevant to an assessment of any claim that might be made about family responsibility by Jane or her aunt. Do family members have responsibility just in virtue of being members of a family? Were we to pursue this line of analysis, a phenomenological approach would require that we assess the ways in which treatment of familial obligation assumes certain models of family life and look for evidence that those patterns existed in the stories. Thus, before a phenomenologist could appropriately rely on an appeal to family obligations in this case, one would need to be clear about the basic meaning of a family and its instantiation in the case example.

In our society, it is tacitly assumed that a family is biologically determined, however, we readily recognise alternative families constructed not on biological but social and psychological bases. Can a biological family not constitute a true 'family' for ethical analysis if family relationships do not meet certain psychological conditions? These are questions that naturally arise for a phenomenologist, because the phenomenological method requires that taken-for-granted beliefs or assumptions, whether they are assumptions within bioethics and philosophy or in ordinary experience, be analysed. Because we are dealing with a text, there is no going beyond the textual evidence. In clinical ethics cases, where the bioethicist functions as an ethics consultant, there is the possibility of interacting directly in order to achieve a different type of evidence. Rather than relying on a health professional's characterisation of a patient's beliefs or attitudes, a phenomenologically trained clinical bioethicist would interview the patient directly. Importantly, the presentation of this case illustrates this phenomenological concern by relying not on a single story but five stories told by five individuals: Jane, Phyllis, the GP, geneticist and oncologist. They are first-person reports, thus illustrating the priority that the case gives to each protagonist as an agent.

Jane is the central character in this story because her situation prompts the conflict of confidentiality and the principle of doing no harm to another patient. She conveys a knowledge about breast cancer that is the product of her own family history, but something that when she was younger was regarded as 'remote to *me*'. While the focus of this case is her breast cancer, she discloses early in her story that her prime concern was 'not being there for my girls'. This fear of every parent illustrates what Alfred Schutz (1971) has termed the *fundamental anxiety*, an anxiety about our finitude. This anxiety drives our actions in the social world and underlies our construction and enactment of projects. This case illustrates how this fundamental anxiety is addressed in advanced technological societies by what Ivan Illich (1976) termed 'medicalization', namely, seeing existential problems as open to technological medical solutions, in this case prophylactic mastectomy.

Jane reported that she had to be 'persuaded' by her husband to see a doctor. Her *angst* motivates him to encourage her to see a doctor. She reported that her husband was optimistic. A newspaper article about genetic testing finally led her to raise the question with her GP. Clearly, she wanted an answer, and she expected an answer with a significant degree of certainty.

Her basic anxiety is not likely to be quelled by the professional assurance of her GP, so a specialist is consulted. She seems to want a technological answer, because she wants her problem to be amenable to human control (Agich 1981).

From the information she received, she believes that she may have inherited a 'rogue' gene from her mother. If she could be tested, then she would have the knowledge she seeks. She says that the 'only problem' is that the test is not definitive. That is why securing information about her mother's relatives is important. It can increase the probability of knowledge about her future and provide a more reliable guide for her decision-making. She seeks out her Aunt Phyllis with whom she has had virtually no contact, because she is so committed to a solution that she is willing to consider prophylactic mastectomy that removes almost the entire breast so as to prevent the development of cancer. She reports, with some hope, that the geneticist told her that there was 'evidence' to show that women who had the operation probably did better than those who followed a regimen of breast examination and mammography. Supported by her husband, she became convinced that this is the solution. 'If I have the operation, then I can stop worrying. I was so fed up with having this gnawing anxiety constantly at the back of my head.' She appears to have made up her mind about a procedure that is disfiguring and has unproven clinical value.

By systematically considering the latent or background meetings that influence decision-making, a phenomenological approach can help us gain a more critical hold on this case. Jane seems motivated by a once-and-for-all fix to her problem. There is no indication that she – or the physicians involved – adequately considered her risk for other cancers besides breast cancer. Apparently, they did not consider the risk of ovarian cancer, which mastectomy does not affect. Jane also exhibits a belief in the certainty of medical knowledge despite the fact that the knowledge of breast-cancer genetics is new and emerging. Not surprisingly, recommendations for procedures such as radical mastectomy can alter over time as can the estimation of risk. New studies suggest that this taken-for-granted focus on breast cancer and mastectomy may be a misplaced response to BRCA (Haber 2002, Kauff et al. 2002, Rebbeck et al. 2002). A phenomenologist would be interested in the way in which various kinds of scientific evidence and clinical judgement are selectively based on individual – be they patient or physician – values and beliefs.

Jane's story raises an additional question. She clearly suffers from anxiety about breast cancer. Does her anxiety need attention as a corollary to the investigation of her prognosis regarding breast cancer? Importantly, the GP and geneticist did not take this up, raising the question of the adequacy of the professional assessments carried out, particularly by the GP. It appeared that the patient, rather than the doctor, defined *the* problem in this case. She came to him with concern about breast cancer and the case became a case *about breast cancer*. Her anxiety was left, as it were, in the shadows. This illustrates another important phenomenological point: all thought and perception displays a Gestalt-like character, namely, there is an object or theme that defines the focal concern, but other elements are horizontal. They define the field or background against which the thematic item stands out and is the focus of attention. Medicine has a long commitment to scientific methodology. There are tests for markers of genetic disease and the practice of genetic diagnosis and counselling relies, sometimes uncritically, on these tests. The clinical project focused on confirming what Jane already believed. This raises a question about informed consent. Had she made up her mind before receiving counselling? Under these circumstances, can she give a fully informed consent? If the answer were affirmative, then a phenomenologist would suggest that we might need to rethink standard understandings of informed consent. In the standard view, informed consent involves a strictly rational decision based on information provided about risks, benefits and alternatives to a proposed treatment. It is a process of decision-making driven by information. It is not guided by desire and values, and only partially shaped by individual beliefs. In this case, however, Jane's decision appeared to be foreshadowed by her uninformed beliefs and values.

Jane herself notes the inadequacy of current genetic testing. Its technological weakness, however, leads her to seek another technological fix, namely, mastectomy, that she, perhaps incorrectly in the light of evidence previously cited, will address her problem with greater certainty. The fact that her husband thinks that mastectomy is a good idea validates her decision to have surgery, but we can ask whether surgery will ultimately quell her anxiety or improve her outcome. Alternatively, were this a case for ethics consultation, a phenomenologically oriented ethics consultant would attempt to ascertain the degree to which Jane's preference for surgery was influenced by her husband's concerns about breast cancer and the potential loss of his wife. Does either of them fully understand that although mastectomy may limit the chance of breast cancer, it might not affect outcome. That is, Jane's life expectancy may not be extended. This concern is not forthrightly addressed in the case.

In Jane's case, her family history provides stronger evidence for a breast-cancer risk than could be provided by direct testing. Current testing yields false negatives, so Jane could not reliably be assured that a negative test result meant that she carried no risk. In similar fashion, the focus of the test is the individual who provides the sample but the results carry implications for family members as well. This points to the essential interconnectedness of human experience. Meanings in the everyday world of life *are* shared. Jane's aunt might have reasons for not wanting to allow her own medical condition to be disclosed to family members based on their past attitudes and behaviour towards her. She does not think that she is close enough emotionally to her family. Genetics, however, points to a close biological connection. The interest in Jane's aunt lies less in her unique medical or biological circumstances than in a shared gene that is strongly associated with breast cancer in her niece, so knowing the family history provides greater predictive power. Families are complex social institutions about which standard assumptions are put to a critical test by genetics. An ethical theory of familial obligations is needed to address the dilemmas that genetic medicine is raising ethically. Such a theory will need to challenge a tacit belief in much of mainstream bioethics, namely, that the fulcrum for analysis is the isolated individual who is protected by a shield of rights. Viewed genetically, none of us is completely isolated.

In thinking about evidence for genetic disease, we need to ask if the presumption that guides Phyllis, the GP and the geneticist, namely, that the test results belong to the individual is really correct? Phyllis presented to the geneticist with the BRCA1 mutation already identified. In this situation, the geneticist says, there is typically a presumption that relatives will be informed, but the geneticist does not believe that geneticists have the authority to contact individuals directly. Jane and Phyllis were referred independently to the geneticist who saw Jane, while a colleague saw Phyllis. Only subsequently did they discover that these patients were related, which created the ethical dilemma for them, namely, that the picture painted by Jane's and Phyllis's situation when taken collectively is much sharper then when regarded independently. Mainstream bioethics might be inclined to argue that Jane's and Phyllis' rights were violated, because a wall was not maintained between the geneticists in the practice. A phenomenologist would argue that such a separation should not be assumed to exist but should be created only if strong ethical argument can be mustered in its defence. As a society, we need to be able to differentiate legitimate from illegitimate uses of medical information, including genetic information. Simply asserting that Phyllis has a right to privacy fails to come to terms with the complex connections that genetic information and knowledge shows exists between individuals. A relational theory of autonomy is clearly needed to begin to address the complex ethical questions that this case poses. The ethical dilemmas involved in this case are also partly structured by the traditional understanding of medical ethics involving a relationship between a physician and an individual patient. Obligations such as confidentiality or informed consent are owed to individuals who are seen in isolation from family/society. This entire framework needs to be reconsidered.

The geneticist points out that in typical cases patients want their family members to know and voluntarily disclose the findings of their testing. Presumably, these individuals feel filial responsibilities that Phyllis, unfortunately, does not acknowledge. This raises the two important questions. First, can the typical focus of obligations on the individual in the physician–patient relationship be sustained as our understanding of disease more fully embraces genetic causation? Second, reliance on private and patient acceptance of familial obligations presumes intact and well-functioning families. Empirical evidence, however, suggests that significant numbers of families are dysfunctional. The same emotional bonds and commitments that create the sense of obligation and commitment toward members of one's family can also create resentment. Jane preserves the very same pattern of behaviour towards Phyllis that Phyllis complains about, namely, Phyllis is taken for granted and approached by Jane only when Jane believes that Phyllis can be of help to her. Jane does not demonstrate gratitude or even much awareness of the care that Phyllis provided for her own mother at the end of her life. Jane did not maintain contact with Phyllis after her mother died, so it would be hard to maintain that Phyllis owed Jane a special obligation based on familial attachment. Phyllis's story is filled with resentment toward her family. It is, of course, impossible to know from the stories whether it is justified but negative feelings are associated with Phyllis's attitudes toward her family. Their presence signals that a stronger case for filial responsibilities will need to contend with such circumstances.

Summary

The strength of a phenomenological approach to the analysis of clinical ethics cases is found in the way the method helps the bioethicist to consciously guide the analysis. By differentiating what is immediately apparent in a case from the latent or background meanings and interpretations, phenomenology helps the bioethicist to select features of the case for analysis. In doing so, phenomenology allows bioethics to be more responsive to the actual ethical problems that emerge in the practice of medicine and to develop an ethical framework that captures the concrete problems of clinical medicine. Phenomenological method also constrains us not to accept uncritically the obvious or apparent aspects of the case, but to seek the best evidence that is available to guide our analysis. It encourages us to be aware of the assumptions that underlie our approach to a case as well as the assumptions of the agents involved in the clinical case.

REFERENCES

Agich, G. J. (1981). The question of technology in medicine. In S. Skousgaard, ed., *Phenomenology and Understanding Human Destiny*. Washington DC: Center for Advanced Research in Phenomenology and University Press of America, 81–92.

(1993). *Autonomy and Long-Term Care*. New York: Oxford University Press, 76–113.

(2004). *Dependence and Autonomy in Old Age*. Cambridge: Cambridge University Press.

Gurwitsch, A. (1978). *The Field of Consciousness*. Pittsburgh: Duquesne University Press.

Haber, D. (2002). Prophylactic oophorectomy to reduce the risk of ovarian and breast cancer in carriers of BRCA mutations. *N Engl J Med*, **346**(21), 1660–2.

Husserl, E. (1969). *Formal and Transcendental Logic* (D. Cairns, tr.). The Hague: Martinus Nijhoff.

(1967). *Ideas: General Introduction to a Pure Phenomenology* (W. R. B. Gibson, tr.). New York: Collier Books.

Illich, I. (1976). *Medical Nemesis: The Expropriation of Health*. New York: Pantheon Books.

Kauff, N. D., Satagopan, J. M., Robson, M. E. *et al.* (2002). Risk-reducing salpingo-oophorectomy in women with BRCA1 or BRCA2 mutation. *N Engl J Med*, **346** (21), 1609–15.

Rebbeck, T. R., Lynch, H. T., Neuhausen, S. L. *et al.* (2002). Prophylactic oophorectomy in carriers of BRCA1 or BRCA2 mutations. *N Engl J Med*, **346**(21), 1616–22.

Schutz, A. (1967). *Phenomenology of the Social World* (G. Walsh and F. Lehnert, trs.). Evanston: Northwestern University Press.

(1971). *Collected Papers. I: The Problem of Social Reality*, ed. M. Natanson. The Hague: Martinus Nijhoff, 226–9.

Schutz, A. and Luckman, T. (1973). *Structures of the Life-World*, (R. M. Zaner and H. T. Englehardt, Jr., trs.). Evanston: Northwestern University Press.

Spiegelberg, H. (1982). *The Phenomenological Movement: A Historical Introduction*, 3rd edn. rev. The Hague: Martinus Nijhoff.

Zaner, R. M. (1973). Reflections on evidence and criticism in the theory of consciousness. In D. Carr and E. S. Casey, eds., *Explorations in Phenomenology*. The Hague: Martinus Nijhoff, 184–207.

BIBLIOGRAPHY

Gurwitsch, A. (1978). *Human Encounters in the Social World*. Pittsburgh: Duquesne University Press.

Husserl, E. (1999). *The Idea of Phenomenology* (L. Hardy, tr.). Dordrecht: Kluwer Academic Publishers.

Schutz, A. (1970). *Reflections on the Problem of Relevance*, ed. R. M. Zaner. New Haven: Yale University Press.

Schutz, A. (1971). *Collected Papers. II: Studies in Social Theory*, ed. A. Brodersen. The Hague: Martinus Nijhoff.

Schutz, A. (1971). *Collected Papers. III: Studies in Phenomenological Philosophy*, ed. I. Schutz. The Hague: Martinus Nijhoff.

13

An empirical approach

Søren Holm

In the analysis of most problems in bioethics, knowledge about the state of the world and our abilities to intervene in it play a significant role. Many ethical problems only emerge when our ability to intervene in the world increases, and it is often important to know in some detail what is possible and what is not. In our ethical arguments we can therefore often discern premises of two kinds: ethical premises and empirical premises.

This means that valid ethical arguments can become false if either of these two kinds of premises is false. If I, for instance, base my analysis of the ethics of communication with persons with terminal illness on the *empirical premise* that most people who are told that they are terminally ill will become severely depressed and will never recover from their depression, I may well reach a quite different *ethical conclusion* than if I base the analysis on the premise that such depression is neither widespread nor permanent.

We can further subdivide empirical premises into three groups, each answering a different kind of ethically relevant question:
1. What is the state of the world?
2. What are our possibilities of intervening in the world?
3. What are the consequences of our interventions?

The first task of an empirical approach to bioethics is therefore to identify the explicit and implicit/enthymematic empirical premises in ethical arguments and try to find out whether they are supported by research findings and theories in the relevant scientific fields. In some cases the knowledge that we need may be biological or biotechnical,[1] in others it may be sociological, anthropological or psychological. It will often be found that our ethical arguments use empirical premises that are not well-substantiated or that are directly contradicted by available research.

An important part of this analysis of empirical premises is an analysis of the quality of the evidence we have for a given proposition. The empirically minded ethicist must therefore possess knowledge about a range of research methodologies in order to be able to read research papers in a suitably critical

Case Analysis in Clinical Ethics, ed. Richard Ashcroft, Anneke Lucassen, Michael Parker, Marian Verkerk, Guy Widdershoven. Published by Cambridge University Press.

way. The mere fact that some research paper supports proposition X is rarely enough to claim that we know X to be the case. He or she must also be well versed in information retrieval from all of the major scientific databases covering medicine, psychology and the social sciences since the relevant information is often not found just by searching within one of these fields.

In some instances we will, however, find that the empirical premises that are used have never been investigated by the relevant scientific field, either because the question that the premise is an answer to has only been raised very recently, or because the question is only of interest within an ethical discourse. The second task of an empirical approach to bioethics is therefore to identify empirical research questions that need to be answered as part of answering important ethical questions.

A possible third task of an empirical approach to bioethics is to give us knowledge about how actors in the healthcare field identify and analyse ethical problems and what their (implicit) ethical framework is. This third task is more contentious than the first two tasks, because it can be argued that how people do in fact reason about ethics has no bearing on how they should or ought to reason about ethics. Pursuing this discussion is far beyond the scope of the present paper, but even if the argument is correct, which I personally doubt (Holm 1997), there are strong pragmatic reasons to be interested in this kind of reasoning. If we want to influence the ethical decision-making of healthcare professionals and patients we need to understand their way of looking at the ethical world if we are to engage them in any kind of reasonable discussion.

If the accounts in the present case had really been first-person accounts of the dilemmas experienced by persons involved in various roles in the testing for BRCA1 they could very well have formed part of the material of a research project into the (ethical) reasoning and decision-making in this context. Such a study could have followed a methodology along the lines of Hallowell *et al.* (1997).

The theory-ladenness of social knowledge

A specific problem may be thought to occur when the research we rely on for our empirical premises is not biological but from the social sciences, because social science research is often much more overtly influenced by theory than is biological research. Now, there are good reasons to believe that all research has to be theory-based and that many seemingly objective biological statements are as theory-laden as statements in the social sciences (Chalmers 1999) but this is probably not enough to dispel the nagging suspicion that many biological scientists or healthcare professionals have that statements based on social science research are inherently more uncertain than firm biological facts. Is this true? And if it is true, is it a serious problem for the use of social-science results as premises in ethical arguments? It is important to distinguish two variants of this critique.

The first variant of this critique points to the inherent time and context dependence of social knowledge. Whereas the substrate of biological research is stable nature,[2] the substrate of social research is the everchanging features of human societies and cultures. Results from research carried out on family dynamics in British families one hundred years ago can no longer be used as accurate descriptions of the modern British family. Social knowledge becomes obsolete; it has a 'sell by date'. If this is true, it does, however, only show that the empirically minded bioethicist should make sure that the social-science-research results he or she relies on are recent and not obsolete. A similar argument could be put forward with regard to the cultural context in which research is performed. Research results from one culture may not easily be transferable to other cultures. But this again only shows that one has to be careful in choosing which research results to rely on. It is also questionable whether these criticisms actually affect all results of social-science research. Although some products of research are fairly specific statements about social reality, other products of research are theoretical frameworks or smaller theory fragments, and it is not clear that these become obsolete or are culturally relative in the same way as the specific statements. Our understanding of the practice of gift-giving and the function of gifts – which is highly relevant to the current case – is, for instance, still very much influenced by theoretical frameworks developed by Bronislaw Malinowski, Franz Boas and Marcel Mauss at the beginning of the 1900s (Malinowski 1922, Boas 1925, Mauss 1954). Whereas the Trobriand society that Malinowski described has changed radically since that time, the underlying analysis of 'the gift' is still mainly the same.

The second variant of the critique is potentially more damaging. It claims that the theory-ladenness of social-science research means that the research results are dangerously subjective. Unless I subscribe to the underlying theory, I have no reason to accept the results as valid. It is again far beyond the scope of this paper to analyse this claim in full, but it is perhaps worth pointing out that all statements about social events are theory-laden, even so-called common-sense statements. Many of our ethical arguments rely on premises about what will happen if certain social structures are changed, or certain social interventions performed, and it is arguably better to use premises where I am aware of their theoretical background, than premises where the theory-ladenness is hidden.

Identifying empirical premises

Let us get back to the case at hand and see whether we can identify the empirical premises that are important for an ethical analysis (Genetic Information 1999).

The following empirical questions of a medical or biotechnical nature play a role for the framing of the problem and possibly also for the choice of the ethically optimal solution:

1. Are there any other sources of informative genetic material than Phyllis?
2. Does the family belong to a subpopulation with known increased frequency of founder mutations?
3. Are there any prognostic or therapeutic differences between BRCA1-related breast cancer and non-BRCA1-related breast cancer (Phillips *et al.* 1999)?
4. Are there any interventions that can decrease breast-cancer risk and/or breast-cancer mortality in BRCA1-mutation carriers (Eeles 2000, Eeles and Powles 2000, Morrow and Gradishar 2002)?
5. Are there any interventions that can decrease ovarian-cancer risk and/or ovarian-cancer mortality in BRCA1-mutation carriers?

There are at least six women in the family, apart from Phyllis, who have had breast or ovarian cancer, and at least one man who is very likely to have had the mutation (the brother of Jane's grandmother).[3] It is quite likely that tissue or blood samples from one or more of these can be found and BRCA1 testing and/or sequencing performed on these samples. Sequencing from fixed tissue samples is probably at the moment not as accurate as sequencing from unfixed samples or fresh tissue, and it is much more complex and costly, but it is still possible (Wong *et al.* 1998, Tobias *et al.* 2000). Pursuing testing/sequencing of other sources of informative genetic material would be even more likely to succeed if the family belonged to a subpopulation with a known increased frequency of founder mutations, since it would then be possible to carry out direct testing for these specific mutations.[4]

If there are other sources of informative genetic material it means that we can help Jane without involving Phyllis and without Jane getting any knowledge about Phyllis.

If the answers to questions 3 or 5 are affirmative then it may well have been rational to test Phyllis for her BRCA1 mutation, even in a situation where she had, a priori, told us that she would not allow the information to be used to help anyone else in her family. If Phyllis's cancer is prognostically or therapeutically different because it is BRCA1-related, or if knowledge of her BRCA1 status can help us to prevent her from developing or dying from ovarian cancer,[5] then the testing is of potential benefit to her (and it was presumably because she had a different perception of the answer to one of these questions than the geneticist that the oncologist initiated testing).[6]

If the answers to questions 3–5 are negative, then it makes little sense to test either Jane or Phyllis.

From the social sciences and psychology we need to look for the answers to the following questions:

1. Are Phyllis's fears that she may be (further) blamed and stigmatised reasonable?

2. Is Phyllis's reaction unusual?
3. What are the likely social and psychological effects on Jane, her husband, their children and the more extended family and kinship of testing if Jane either is or is not a carrier of the BRCA1 mutation?

If Phyllis's fears are well-founded we are, in effect, asking her to sacrifice part of her well-being in order to secure benefits for someone else. In this case we do not have sufficient information about the relationship between Phyllis and her kin to make any very firm statements about what the effects would be if the kin became aware that Phyllis was carrying the BRCA1 mutation. At a more general level we know that stigma (i.e. the identification of someone as flawed, discredited or spoiled (Goffman 1963))[7] often does attach to chronic illness and also to known or suspected carriers of genetic diseases (Charmaz 2000). Stigma may even attach to healthy heterozygous carriers of recessive disorders. It is thus, at the very least, not unreasonable that Phyllis fears further stigmatisation.

It is also important to know that Phyllis is not unusual in not wanting to share information with family members. Studies show that daughters and other female relatives of persons with breast cancer are often frustrated in their attempts to get information from the person with the cancer, even in those cases where the affected person is their mother (Chalmers and Thomson 1996, Chalmers et al. 1996). This makes it considerably more difficult to conceptualise Phyllis purely as an irrational and embittered old spinster.

Phyllis's reaction is also explainable in another way through an analysis based on theories about the nature and function of gifts. It is a central feature of the system of gifts as it works between social equals that a gift has to be reciprocated at some later time by a gift of similar value. Not reciprocating is a serious matter that displays disdain for the original gift giver or mere callousness. In this family this process has apparently broken down a long time ago, at least seen from Phyllis's perspective. She believes that she has given her mother and sister gifts of considerable value, by having cared for them when they were ill, but she has never received anything back. And on top of this, she is now being asked to give another gift to her family!

With regard to the effects on Jane and her family we know that genetic testing for BRCA1 mutations is not sociologically and psychologically unproblematic, but we also know that it seldom leads to any major social or psychological problems if the family unit in which it is done is stable. BRCA1 testing and the reception of the result may not solve as many problems, and make decision-making easier, as Jane may expect, but it is unlikely to cause her major distress (Lodder et al. 1999, Reichelt et al. 1999).

What about Jane and her husband's two girls if Jane eventually has the test; should they be told of the test result if it is positive, and if so when? If Jane has the BRCA1 mutation each of her daughters has a fifty-per-cent risk of having inherited it, and if the moral arguments support disclosure between Phyllis and Jane, they surely support disclosure between Jane and her daughters. Jane's daughters are currently only 7 and 9 years old and it may not be the right time to communicate with them about cancer risk, although it may well become necessary if Jane chooses to have a bilateral prophylactic mastectomy. We know surprisingly little about the effects on children of being given information about genetic risk even though studies indicate that around half of all parents tested for BRCA1/2 mutations will inform their children about the test result (Tercyak *et al.* 2001). This lack of information was pointed out some years ago (Michie and Martean 1996) but the call for further research seems to have been largely unheeded. This means that we lack important empirical premises relevant for two kinds of arguments: arguments about if and when children should be told about genetic risk; and arguments about whether children should ever be tested for adult-onset genetic disorders. In the literature it is for instance mentioned that 'such testing could cause serious harms, including damage to the child's self-esteem and distortion of the family's perception of the child' (de Wert 1998: 46) but it is surely an empirically answerable question how frequent and how severe such harms are.

Men: the forgotten group in genetic counselling

In one of the Sherlock Holmes stories a key piece of evidence used by the great detective is 'the dog that didn't bark' and in the current case there is also a curious absence that, once noted, may help us to raise new and interesting questions about the case. This absence is the specific lack of interest in poor Uncle George, and in general in the few men that are mentioned by the interlocutors in the case.

Uncle George has a fifty-per-cent risk of being a carrier of the BRCA1 mutation in the family and this puts him at an increased risk of breast cancer, prostate cancer and colon cancer (Struewing *et al.* 1997), but it also puts his two children at a twenty-five-per-cent risk of carrying the mutation, i.e. exactly the same risk as Jane's two children prior to any testing of Jane. Why doesn't George figure much more prominently in the case? He should at least have had some mention in the geneticist's story because the geneticist will know about George's risk from drawing up the family tree.

For the empirically knowledgeable ethicist the absence of George is worrying but not really surprising. In Western societies women are the ones who are mainly responsible for the social maintenance of family ties, including the social maintenance of the family genealogy. Women are 'the genetic housekeepers for the kinship' (Richards 1996, Stacey 1996). 'Genetic' problems in families will therefore mainly be discussed by, and seen as problems by, the women in the family (Rees and Bath 2000). This is reinforced by the asymmetric contribution to human reproduction (i.e. the empirical fact that only women are pregnant) and also leads to a focus on women in genetic counselling. When, as in this case, we are furthermore dealing with a gene that increases the risk of cancer in a highly symbolic female body part, everything is set for a scene where males are likely to be written out of the script (McAllister *et al.* 1998). Any proper resolution of the case must therefore write the men back in.

The absence of the male perspective may in this case hide one possible way of resolving the problem without going against Phyllis's expressed preferences. We know very little about Uncle George from the case but we have one piece of positive information and one piece of negative information that might be relevant. The positive information is that Uncle George knows where Phyllis lives and we can perhaps assume that he has kept some kind of contact with her, and may even know that she has had breast cancer. The negative information is that Phyllis does not mention Uncle George in her complaints about her family; it may therefore be that she has a more neutral relation to him than to her sister. Why not ask Jane to ask Uncle George to come to genetic counselling? If it becomes clear that he knows about Phyllis's breast cancer, then he may be able to ask Phyllis to have a genetic test in order to help him and his children.

Some further observations on the role of the counsellor

It is usually claimed that genetic counselling should be non-directive, i.e. that it should not be prescriptive either with regard to testing or non-testing or with regard to the response to a given test result. It is interesting to note that in this case the geneticist openly admits that 'my colleague has tried hard to suggest to Phyllis that it would be in the interest of her family to disclose, but she just doesn't see it as in her interest. She feels that she would be blamed and stigmatised'. Why does the idea of non-directive counselling not hold true here? Why does the counsellor believe that he or she knows what it would be best for Phyllis to do, and why does he or she feel justified in trying hard to persuade Phyllis?

We know from a number of studies that genetic counselling is directive, despite the stated policy of non-directiveness (Marteau *et al.* 1994, Bartels *et al.* 1997, Michie *et al.* 1997, Sagi *et al.* 2001) but it is seldom as overtly directive as described here. The case actually describes the dilemma faced by the genetic counsellor very accurately (as we have seen above). It is in all probability in the interest of Phyllis's family to get the information about Phyllis's genetic test, but Phyllis does not see it as in her interest and it is probably not in her interest (unless we claim that she has an interest in doing the morally right thing). If the counsellor was mainly interested in doing what is best for Phyllis she should probably have supported her in non-disclosure. What this case shows therefore is that genetic counsellors do not see the welfare of the patient/client or even the narrow family unit as their only consideration. Taking into account the interests of parties other than the patient/client can be supported on moral grounds (as it has in many of the other chapters in the book), but many of those arguments will support directive counselling in a wide range of circumstances where genetic counsellors would traditionally counsel non-directively.

Another conflict that seems to be hidden under the surface of this case is not a directly ethical conflict but an interprofessional one. Our current possibilities within cancer genetics are relatively new, the first cancer gene being identified in 1985 (the retinoblastoma gene). The possibilities increase rapidly and cancer genetics is therefore a growth industry that will employ many people in the future, but who will these people be? Will they be geneticists, genetic counsellors or oncologists?[8] This is a question with important ethical aspects, since it is clearly the case that patients in this new field should be offered good counselling services. But what kinds of counsellors are best? To answer that question we need an answer to the prior question of what counselling is supposed to achieve, but when we have that answer we still need empirical evidence with regard to what kind of counsellors are best suited to achieving the desired goal. We know that different groups of healthcare professionals counsel in different ways (Marteau *et al.* 1994), and we also know that patients prefer different kinds of counsellors in different situations (Hofferbert *et al.* 2000, Audrain *et al.* 1998), but we still know next to nothing about how different counsellors and/or counselling styles affect the decision-making of the patients. We do not, for instance, know whether non-directive counselling and directive counselling actually lead to different outcomes with regard to patient decisions, or even whether patients can differentiate between non-directive and directive counsellors.

Resource allocation

A final area where the empirically oriented bioethicist can add significantly to the analysis of the case is when we move the discussion from the individual case to the broader issue of resource allocation. A case like this does not occur in isolation: it occurs within the context of a healthcare system with specific funding mechanisms and specific resource constraints. We are unable here to analyse this in depth, partly because such an analysis would have to include a discussion of the effects of the contested patent status of the BRCA1 and BRCA2 genes in order to be complete and that is far beyond the scope of this chapter. It is, however, important to note that BRCA1 testing is currently limited by resource constraints in the UK, both with regard to volume and the methods used. This means that we could ask whether these constraints are just, and to answer that question we would need empirical information about what is offered to other patients in a similar situation, what the cost/benefit, cost/utility or cost/effectiveness ratios are for the different available methods of BRCA1 testing, as well as information about non-economic factors restricting access to BRCA1 testing and counselling.

Conclusion

This chapter has shown how different kinds of results from empirical research are crucial for our understanding of the present case, and for many of the ethical arguments that are relevant in the resolution of the case.

It has also shown that just the analysis of one single case, such as this one, uncovers many areas where more empirical research is needed.

NOTES

1 As in the current case where an important premise setting up the whole dilemma is that 'it is only practical to carry out a presymptomatic test in an unaffected woman if a mutation has already been identified' – this is not a logical truth but an empirical statement based on our current knowledge about BRCA1 mutations and our current methods for detecting and interpreting them.

2 But note that 'nature' also changes. The *Staphylococcus aureus* that bothers us today is not the same as the *Staph. aureus* of forty years ago.

3 He is not marked as dead on the family tree but I will assume that he is, otherwise we could just ask him for a blood sample.

4 Many other groups than Ashkenazi Jews have a limited number of founder mutations in BRCA1.

5 It is interesting to note that this case almost exclusively focuses on breast cancer, although BRCA1 mutations also increase the risk of ovarian cancer, a form of cancer with a considerably higher mortality rate than breast cancer.

6 It is interesting to note that Jane has the impression from her genetic counselling that 'there was evidence to show that women like me who had this operation [prophylactic mastectomy] probably did better than women who just examined themselves and had mammograms'. This seems to indicate that the counsellor may also believe that knowing your BRCA1 status gives you valuable information that may help you to decide how to act.

7 Note that 'stigma' is another very useful theoretical construct from the social sciences that has proven durable over time, even if the concrete context of Goffman's original research has long since changed.

8 And even within the group of oncologists there may be further battles between surgical, medical and radiotherapy-oriented oncologists.

REFERENCES

Audrain, J., Rimer, B., Cella, D. *et al.* (1998). Genetic counseling and testing for breast–ovarian cancer susceptibility: what do women want? *J Clin Oncol*, **16**(1), 133–8.

Bartels, D. M., LeRoy, B. S., McCarthy, P. and Caplan, A. L. (1997). Nondirectiveness in genetic counseling: a survey of practitioners. *Am J Med Gen*, **72**(2), 172–9.

Boas, F. (1925). *Contributions to the Ethnology of the Kwakiutl*. New York: Columbia University Press.

Chalmers, A. F. (1999). *What is This Thing Called Science?*, 3rd edn. Buckingham: Open University Press.

Chalmers, K. and Thomson, K. (1996). Coming to terms with the risk of breast cancer: perceptions of women with primary relatives with breast cancer. *Qualitat Health Res*, **6**, 256–82.

Chalmers, K., Thomson, K. and Degner, L. F. (1996). Information, support and communication needs of women with a family history of breast cancer. *Cancer Nursing*, **19**, 204–13.

Charmaz, K. (2000). Experiencing chronic illness. In G. L. Albrecht, R. Fitzpatrick and S. C. Scrimshaw, eds., *The Handbook of Social Studies in Health and Medicine*. London: Sage, 277–92.

Eeles, R. A. (2000). Future possibilities in the prevention of breast cancer: intervention strategies in BRCA1 and BRCA2 mutation carriers. *Breast Cancer Res*, **2**(4), 283–90.

Eeles, R. A., and Powles, T. J. (2000). Chemoprevention options for BRCA1 and BRCA2 mutation carriers. *J Clin Oncol*, **18**(21Suppl.); 93S–99S.

Genetic testings for Cancer: The surgeon's critical role. (1999). *J Am Coll Surg* **188**(1), 74–93. This comprises the following consecutive articles: Vogelstien, B. Familial colon cancer. 74–9; Weber, B. L. Familial breast cancer. 79–86; Greely, H. T. Ethical and legal issues associated with genetic testing. 86–9; and Peterson, G. Clinical cancer genetics 1998 (what's available to you in your practice). 89–93.

Goffman, E. (1963). *Stigma*. Englewood Cliffs, New Jersey: Prentice Hall.

Hallowell, N., Murton, F., Statham, H., Green, J. M. and Richards, M. P. M. (1997). Women's need for information before attending genetic counselling for familial breast or ovarian cancer: a questionnaire, interview, and observational study. *BMJ*, **314**(7076), 281–3.

Hofferbert, S., Worringen, U., Backe, J., *et al.* (2000). Simultaneous interdisciplinary counseling in German breast/ovarian cancer families: first experience with patient perceptions, surveillance behavior and acceptance of genetic testing. *Genetic Counseling*, **11**(2), 127–46.

Holm, S. (1997). *Ethical Problems in Clinical Practice: The Ethical Reasoning of Health Care Professionals*. Manchester: Manchester University Press.

Lodder, L. N., Frets, P. G., Trijsburg, R. W. *et al.* (1999). Presymptomatic testing for BRCA1 and BRCA2: how distressing are the pre-test weeks? *J Med Gen*, **36**(12), 906–13.

Malinowski, B. (1922). *Argonauts of the Western Pacific: An Account of Native Enterprise and Adventure in the Archipelagoes of Melanesian New Guinea*. London: Routledge.

Marteau, T. M., Drake, H. and Bobrow, M. (1994). Counselling following diagnosis of fetal abnormality: the differing approaches of obstetricians, clinical geneticists, and genetic nurses. *J Med Gen*, **31**(11), 864–7.

Mauss, M. (1954). *The Gift. Forms and Functions of Exchange in Archaic Societies.* London: Cohen & West. [Originally Published in French 1923–4.]

McAllister, M. F., Evans, D. G. R., Ormiston, W., and Daly, P. (1998). Men in breast cancer families: a preliminary study of awareness and experience. *J Med Gen*, **35**(9), 739–44.

Michie, S. and Marteau, T. M. (1996). Predictive genetic testing in children: the need for psychological research. *Br J Health Psychol*, **1**, 3–14.

Michie, S., Bron, F., Bobrow, M. and Marteau, T. M. (1997). Nondirectiveness in genetics counseling: an empirical study. *Am J Human Gen*, **60**(1), 40–7.

Morrow, M. and Gradishar, W. (2002). Recent developments: breast cancer. *BMJ*, **324**, 410–14.

Phillips, K. A., Andrulis, I. L. and Goodwin, P. J. (1999). Breast carcinomas arising in carriers of mutations in BRCA1 or BRCA2: are they prognostically different? *J Clin Oncol*, **17**(11), 3653–63.

Rees, C. E. and Bath, P. A. (2000). The information needs and source preferences of women with breast cancer and their family members: a review of the literature published between 1988 and 1998. *J Adv Nursing*, **31**(4), 833–41.

Reichelt, J. G., Dahl, A. A., Heimdal, K. and Møller, P. (1999). Uptake of genetic testing and pre-test levels of mental distress in Norwegian families with known BRCA1 mutations. *Dis Markers*, **15**(1–3), 139–43.

Richards, M. (1996). Families, kinship and genetics. In T. Marteau and M. Richards, eds., *The Troubled Helix: Social and Psychological Implications of the New Human Genetics.* Cambridge: Cambridge University Press, 249–73.

Sagi, M., Meiner, V., Reshef, N., Dagan, J. and Zlotogora, J. (2001). Prenatal diagnosis of sex chromosome aneuploidy: possible reasons for high rates of pregnancy termination. *Prenatal Diag*, **21**(6), 461–5.

Stacey, M. (1996). The new genetics: a feminist view. In T. Marteau and M. Richards, eds., *The Troubled Helix: Social and Psychological Implications of the New Human Genetics.* Cambridge: Cambridge University Press, 331–49.

Struewing, J. P., Hartge, P., Wacholder, S. *et al.* (1997). The risk of cancer associated with specific mutations of BRCA1 and BRCA2 among Ashkenazi Jews. *N Engl J Med*, **336**, 1401–7.

Tercyak, K. P., Hughes, C., Main, D., *et al.* (2001). Parental communication of BRCA1/2 genetic test results to children. *Patient Ed Counsel*, **42**, 213–24.

Tobias, D. H., Eng, C., McCurdy, L. D. *et al.* (2000). Founder BRCA1 and 2 mutations among a consecutive series of Ashkenazi Jewish ovarian cancer patients. *Gynecol Oncol*, **78**(2), 148–51.

De Wert, G. (1998). Ethics of predictive DNA testing for hereditary breast and ovarian cancer. *Patient Ed Counsel*, **35**: 43–52.

Wong, C., DiCioccio, R. A., Allen, H. J., Werness, B. A. and Piver, M. S. (1998). Mutations in BRCA1 from fixed, paraffin-embedded tissue can be artifacts of preservation. *Cancer Gen Cytogen*, **107**(1), 21–7.

14

Response to ethical dissections of the case

Anneke Lucassen

As the author of the case scenario, I have been asked to describe my thoughts about and reactions to the different ethical treatments of the case. What is it like to work together with a bunch of ethicists? (What is a good collective noun for ethicists: a consideration of ethicists? A quandary, or perhaps a cerebration of ethicists?) I have been fascinated, intrigued, intimidated and impressed in equal measure but above all, I have found the experience immensely enjoyable. I would like to respond to some of the issues raised in the different analyses here and hope that the reader, who has acquired this book to tap into a rich seam of ethical expertise, will bear with an often personal, sometimes perhaps a bit touchy, reaction to some of the comments.

Have these different ethical approaches helped me in deciding how to manage this case? Yes, I think they have. My decision on whether to disclose Phyllis's result may not have altered but it is now more considered and I am clearer as to why I would choose to do so. I have also changed my mind about certain aspects of the case. This is, of course, not to say that I now think there is a 'correct' answer to the dilemma. I agree with Gillon that there is no 'correct' answer to a true moral dilemma but I am clearer in my own mind why I would opt for one solution rather than the other and I feel this clarity is a result of hearing and reading the different perspectives raised in these chapters.

One of the things that drew me into the speciality of clinical genetics was that its practice differs from the standard medical consultation. The focus is very much on families and how a particular condition affects that *family* rather than the more focused one-to-one of the traditional medical relationship. We have time in the 45- to 60-minute consultation to find out more about family stories and interactions. Although many families are happy to share genetic information, tensions, difficulties or lack of communication within families are commonplace and genetic information can carry a particular stigma for individuals within that family. While the case discussed in this book may be an extreme example of non-communication, variants of this

Case Analysis in Clinical Ethics, ed. Richard Ashcroft, Anneke Lucassen, Michael Parker, Marian Verkerk, Guy Widdershoven. Published by Cambridge University Press.

are seen in the everyday working lives of clinical genetics departments. Furthermore, today's medical profession is particularly aware of issues relating to consent and confidentiality: recent public enquiries and ongoing court cases add to an awareness that appropriate respect of each should be seen to be done. I do not think that clinical genetic professionals would have very different views on consent and confidentiality than other medical professionals, but in dealing with the family group they may have the tensions that these issues can create within families more acutely focused for them.

Clinical genetics professionals (by this I mean the doctors, nurses and counsellors working in a clinical genetics team) would, I think, be divided on how to manage this case. Many would have in-house facilities for discussing these sorts of dilemmas (such as the ones facilitated by Mike Parker in Oxford) or would bring their case to a national forum such as the Genethics Club (www.genethicsclub.org). Consultation and debate at this kind of interface can be enormously helpful in unravelling the knots of a particular case and also in formulating and developing guidelines for future practice. For example, one of the early cases we discussed with Mike Parker in the Oxford Genetics Service was what to do if a by-product of genetic testing revealed that paternity had been misattributed (Lucassen and Parker 2001). Most of the research in this area showed that genetic workers favoured 'fudging' the issue by lying about the results of genetic tests. Professional guidelines and legal cases did not clarify the situation. There was heated debate around the subject and opinions remain divided. Although an emerging theme seems to be that such possibilities should be raised at the outset rather than dealt with when they are discovered (Human Genetics Commission 2002), it is not clear how much practice has altered in this area. That is to say: are genetic workers now more likely to say in some shape or form, 'this test could reveal that you are not the father of little Johnny'? My somewhat anecdotal evidence would suggest that the majority might still have a tendency to fudge the issues.

In practice, communicating this sort of information is tricky; we feel awkward about it and it is because here the 'medical facts' are inextricably entwined with the emotions and everyday life of the family that clinical genetics becomes more complex than simply a service to supply information to families. Ashcroft comments on the inextricability of genetic testing and counselling from its social context and I agree. Interestingly, the term 'counselling' is enough to put some people off their appointment: 'I don't want any counselling, just the genetic test please' is a reaction the clinical service often meets. As a consequence the term 'genetic advice' is sometimes used, but this may seem to deny that the professionals are drawn in; we have our own preconceived ideas (as Agich and others point out). We cannot be truly non-directive and most of us are honest enough to know that this is so (Clarke 1991). We might aim to be as neutral as possible and to hide our own views, say, on the rights or wrongs of termination of pregnancy, but we would know that our views will probably not be entirely hidden, and that silence on a subject may be as directive as expressing an opinion.

Do the authors arrive at the same conclusions regarding this acute dilemma? Not surprisingly they do not, and although not all authors commit themselves in 'taking a stance' the impression gained from reading the chapters is that there is a roughly three-way split. Gillon and Campbell would not disclose, Holm probably would not; I get the sense Agich would not either. Savulescu definitely would as would Parker and Hurwitz; Ashcroft, Verkerk and Widdershoven do not commit either way. So, it is clearly not an easy case to resolve and I am reassured by that! I have not missed something obvious that any self-respecting ethicist would have seen immediately.

I had predicted when embarking on this project that some approaches would appeal to me more than others, and this was so but not along the lines I had thought. For example, I had anticipated that the empirical approach would appeal since it relied so strongly on evidence and facts and seemed very rational, yet this did not particularly help me, partly because there is so little empirical evidence in this area. Some of the empirical evidence chosen by Holm is now outdated and some of the research he quotes is conflicted by other studies. For example, male carriers of BRCA1 are not thought to be at increased risk of breast cancer. Any increased risk in prostate cancer is likely to be very small, if at all, and the small increased risk of colon cancer is seen mainly in women carriers and thought to be at least in part due to wrongly diagnosed ovarian cancer (Brose *et al.* 2002, Thompson and Easton 2002, Meijers-Heijboer *et al.* 2004). To me, it seemed the empirical evidence presented was biased, or presented only part of the (at-present-uncertain) picture so the whole approach became less relevant. To bemoan the lack of interest in 'poor old Uncle George' and portray the genetics services as wilfully ignoring the men in the family (Holm) seems obtuse. Of course, he would be an avenue to explore, yet this case was chosen specifically because it did not allow this option. Men are not 'the forgotten group' in genetic counselling. Holm's suggested solution of 'just asking [a male relative] for a blood sample' has some serious ethical, if not practical, objections: those of approaching a member of the family who has not been referred to any of the specialists involved in the case and who has not asked for any contact.

Other approaches also seem to criticise the case for not finding a solution lying outside the story. Perhaps I should have made it clearer that the genetics services would have explored any possible alternative solutions to the dilemma. For example, Agich says 'there is no indication she or her physicians adequately considered the risk for other cancers'. In reality, of course, they would have but the story was specifically constructed around a case of breast-cancer risk! Agich also questions the adequacy of professional assessment in not pursuing Jane's anxiety. Again, of course, this would be a standard part of assessment and indeed most clinical genetics units would have a dedicated clinical psychologist who sees patients considering prophylactic surgery. It is simply not possible in one chapter to describe all the interactions of the different members of the family and in any case the story was about Jane and Phyllis, the two patients. I found these approaches less helpful because they seemed to be saying 'this is not really a dilemma because you've missed something' or 'it can all be solved by a third way'.

I might have also predicted that the finer academic machinations of post-structuralist ethics would go over my head, but I found this one of the more appealing approaches. I was intrigued by the approach of destabilising the taken-for-granted assumptions that all information about the body belongs to the patient. Genetic information is text yet we also think of it as the body to which it belongs and confidentiality is not necessarily a prerequisite for trust (Withers). Often genetic conditions have certain characteristics on display so these cannot be kept confidential. If Phyllis had, say, achondroplasia, her genetic-test result would be public knowledge. The dilemma would be different because the altered genetic code can be inferred from observing her walking down the street: not all genetic information is therefore necessarily confidential information. As Ashcroft says 'confidentiality is a form of managing the boundary between secret self and public face'.

A bit about the characters

Although the case scenario is based on real cases, ultimately the author (as Hurwitz points out) was the clinical geneticist, so Jane and Phyllis, the GP and the oncologist were all brought into being by a clinical geneticist. Did that introduce bias? Inevitably, some, yes, but I have tried to write the case from the point of view of the individual characters. I am also a mother, an aunt, a sister and come from a family that sometimes functions poorly. I feel qualified to take more than just the position of the clinical geneticist. In many ways, the story of Phyllis is more influenced by my memories of an elderly aunt than it is by my medical experience, and in many ways the story of the GP is influenced by many years of close friendships with several of them.

But since I penned the characters I also want to say something about how I saw them. Contrary to what a lot of the chapters assumed, I have a lot of sympathy for Phyllis. She is indeed grumpy, isolated and defensive, but I do not suspect her of malice. I do not think she really understood the huge difference that her result could make to Jane, and if genetics services were in a position to do so, then 'forced mediation' (Hurwitz and Gillon) may well have convinced her that Jane should have known of her result. She had simply not been asked in the right way (partly because her doctors were so nervous of raising the issue of breaching confidentiality). I see Phyllis as having been in a corner, but not necessarily wanting to be there. She might have been coaxed out gently, if only someone in the family would have seen who she really is. In doing so she might have found the world outside her corner a happier place to be. I agree with Gillon then, that my hope is also that Phyllis will offer a way out of the dilemma. When Campbell writes 'the temptations of the doctors to bully her into [disclosing her result] or to do it behind her back are utterly misplaced' this seems far removed from how such clinical situations appear to me in practice. Phyllis should not be bullied and as Gillon says: 'a discussion with Phyllis without bullying or browbeating ought to take place'. I agree with Withers that trust is not necessarily 'bound up in maintaining confidentiality' and that 'I need to trust the physician to do the right thing despite my insistence that she do the wrong thing'.

Many chapters assume that Jane went to see her aunt Phyllis knowing that she had breast cancer or hoping to get something from her. In fact I had in mind a much more open-ended situation. When the geneticist first saw Jane she did not know about Aunt Phyllis either, but suggested contact with her as she might have had more information about other relatives that Jane did not know about, for example, the branch that had emigrated to Australia. Jane was rather bewildered by her aunt's grumpiness, being to a large extent ignorant of her previous generation's feud. It did not really occur to her that her aunt might have cancer and not tell her about it. Although a terrifying prospect for Jane, cancer does not have the stigma that it does for Phyllis.

Then the poor oncologist – he gets a very bad press and this is not at all how I had seen him. He is accused of 'professional misconduct' (Ashcroft) and incurring 'raised eyebrows' (Campbell) but I do not believe this to be the case. It is unusual for oncologists to send off samples for BRCA testing, but not inappropriate. Indeed one could question whether consenting for the benefit of relatives should be his job since none of these relatives are his patients. He had sincere and reasonable motives for taking the sample – the risk of ovarian cancer for one was clarified by the result, and Phyllis may well benefit from a prophylactic oophorectomy both for ovarian cancer and future breast-cancer risk. Many chapters assume that because he ordered a genetic test he should have discussed the implications for other family members. He may well have done so but Phyllis did not remember these discussions because they were at the time of her diagnosis and they did not seem relevant to her then. Many people do not recall all aspects of a medical consultation, or all the nuances of what they have consented to. Furthermore, although genetic testing is not yet that prevalent, there are many non-genetic tests that, in effect, make a genetic diagnosis. For example, routine antenatal screening by ultrasound may make a genetic diagnosis. Most information leaflets or consent procedures for this test would not discuss the possible implications for relatives. Biochemical neonatal screening can make a genetic diagnosis; currently there would be little if any counselling up front on the implications for relatives. Neonatal screening is set to expand to genetic testing for cystic fibrosis and haemoglobinopathies for the entire UK population. I doubt whether each parent will be counselled prior to testing that the result may have implications for relatives. Practical difficulties are, of course, no defence, and arguments could be made that this should be done, but certainly the oncologist would not have been acting outside the realms of current routine practice.

Consent for disclosure as a precondition to testing

I have changed my mind about certain things. I now disagree with my earlier stance that a precondition of taking a blood sample should be to have agreement on the sharing of the result with relatives. I agree with Widdershoven and others that 'responsibility towards their relatives might not be promoted by just demanding consent at the outset'. Such a precondition may simply ensure that people with doubts about disclosing results to family members miss out on genetic testing. So, such a precondition may prevent the genetic department from feeling the dilemma, but it does not solve the situation. While we would always aim to get consent, if we do not obtain it, it does not necessarily follow that all trust will be lost in the medical profession, if in rare circumstances confidentiality is breached. Although Parker's chapter suggests that such a precondition should be an important part of a genetics-centre policy, I am also grateful to him for the analogy that helped to change my mind. A person with epilepsy will be advised that they should not continue to drive and the vehicle-licensing authority (DVLA) in the UK will be informed, hopefully with their consent. However, if they do not consent, confidentiality could be breached because of the risk to others. If a neurologist were to say 'I will only see you as a patient if you consent to me informing the DVLA about you' this prerequisite would be seen as unreasonable and not conducive to obtaining a greater level of consent to such disclosure. Similarly, a genetics service may hope that family members will agree to the sharing of their genetic information where relevant but cannot insist on it as a prerequisite to being seen. Equally, if a person does not give consent when asked, there may be special circumstances in which that person's confidentiality might be breached.

Some technical aspects of the case

I enjoyed the chapters of Agich and Campbell but, unfortunately, both had misunderstood some of the genetic complexities and thus their conclusions may well have been different had the genetic issues been clearer for them.

These misunderstandings are likely to be representative of many, since the field is complicated and difficult to convey clearly in one case history. Campbell describes the dilemma Jane faces as whether to have a mastectomy or not. This clearly is a dilemma but not the subject of this book. Jane has decided, after long and hard thinking, that she will have this operation as she knows she is at increased risk. The dilemma is that the clinicians have a piece of information that Jane does not know about, namely that she could have a highly accurate, quick genetic test that has a fifty-per-cent chance of showing her that she does not need this surgery.

Campbell says 'would all this change for Jane if the doctors decided to breach confidentiality and test her for the rogue gene associated with her aunt's cancer? Here the science is complicated, but, as I understand it, considerable uncertainty would remain, unless it were definitely shown that Jane had the same rogue gene'. In fact, it is the other way round: if Jane could be shown *not* to have the same rogue gene as Phyllis then there would be considerable *certainty* that a mastectomy is ill-advised. Campbell therefore sees the disclosure of Phyllis's result as leading to only more uncertainty; he weighs this against a loss of trust in the physician–patient relationship and (perhaps not surprisingly) comes down against disclosure. Where would he have come down if he had understood the science differently?

Agich recommends fudging the issues for Jane – to advise against surgery and not disclose the source of the physician's information. Does he mean this advice to come after an illicit predictive test? Or would he just advise against it anyway, in which case he seems to be ignoring mounting evidence of benefit (Hartmann et al. 1999, Frost et al. 2000, Meijers-Heijboer et al. 2001). Agich says that 'Jane appears to have made up her mind about a procedure that is disfiguring and has unproven clinical value'. Would he recommend she do nothing? There is also no evidence that mammography or breast examination reduces mortality from breast cancer in Jane's age group, and a theoretical risk of inducing a breast cancer by the radiation in repeated mammography (summarized in Lucassen et al. 2001); Would he also dismiss this as an option for her? There is very little clear evidence for surveillance or preventative options in cancer genetics. This lack of evidence does not usually mean that studies have shown no benefit, but rather that there have been insufficient studies to prove benefit.

Agich says that phenomenology seeks 'to obtain the best evidence that is available to guide our analysis' – these are laudable aims but not entirely apparent in the choice of evidence presented. He suggests that 'new studies suggest that this taken-for-granted focus on breast cancer and mastectomy may be a misplaced response to BRCA (Haber 2002, Kauff et al. 2002, Rebbeck et al. 2002)'. These quoted studies do indeed talk about prophylactic oophorectomy (PO) as risk-reducing measures for BRCA1 carriers but they do not say that mastectomy is misplaced! It is an additional prophylactic measure to consider, but the breast cancer risk reduction from PO is much smaller than through mastectomy (approximately fifty per cent versus ninety-five per cent summarised in Morrow and Gradishar 2002). He concludes: 'Jane's decision appeared to be foreshadowed by her uninformed beliefs and values.' Why does he think they are uninformed? In fact, Jane is more informed about the pros and cons of prophylactic mastectomy in her situation than most surgeons prepared to do the operation. She has weighed up the limited evidence and the uncertainties and decided that this represents the best option for her.

Anxiety in the medical profession

Recent years have seen a fundamental shift in the doctor–patient relationship. Patients (clients) are seen more as consumers. As Ashcroft points out, the ethics of power might also include the patient as ultimate consumer. What the patient wants must be complied with for fear of being sued. The wake of the UK Alder Hey and Bristol enquiries has resulted in a nervousness and wariness of and by the medical profession. 'Are we doing it right, according to the law?' has in some cases become more important than 'does my patient trust me?'. The medical profession is becoming increasingly cautious and, as Withers says, 'something important and good can be lost to caution'. The new Human Tissue Bill in the UK (which was going through Parliament at the time of writing) is likely to make it a criminal offence to hold a biological sample without consent (previously this might have been a professional offence). Holders of such samples may therefore decide to discard them since the penalty resulting from a lack of diagnosis in the future or a benefit for family members (or future family members) is smaller than the penalty for holding a sample that may not have adequate consent. This new bill may also, it seems, directly oppose the 'firm legal advice' that Gillon received and specifically prohibit disclosure of Phyllis's test result without her consent. Like Gillon, in practice, I would feel inclined to go in the opposite direction of this new legal advice but unlike him I would disclose Phyllis's test result. Gillon uses casuistry to argue that if Phyllis's results were locked in her safe in her flat, no-one would advocate breaking into her flat to steal them for the benefit of Jane. I would agree with this, but it is exactly because Phyllis's result is in the hands of the clinical geneticist, who is also looking after Jane, that the dilemma is different from the flat-safe dilemma.

Clinical practice

This case is unusual in that it is rather acute and we cannot escape from the dilemma by waiting for things possibly to resolve by themselves. Often we would suggest or encourage family communication to see whether this resolves any issues of 'non-disclosure' but in many cases we would not hear back from the family. Jane may not have come back to the genetics service, but gone instead straight to a surgeon, and explained that there was no genetic testing possible and asked for a prophylactic mastectomy. (And in answer to Hurwitz's question: yes, such surgeons could be found with relative ease. They may or may not write to the genetics service beforehand.) In other cases the 'non-disclosure' may occur in families with conditions that are not treatable or preventable, for example Huntington's disease, and there may therefore be less of a time pressure to come up with a solution. A result in one person may be withheld, thus denying others an accurate predictive test. We might encourage communication with other family members (possibly directive, but in the belief that someone should at least be given the choice as to whether or not to test) but have no way of knowing how often this does or does not take place. Some research has shown that it does not in a significant number of cases (Julian-Reynier 2000) and an in-house survey revealed about twenty cases of apparent non-disclosure in our department over a one-year period.

I ended the geneticist story by saying 'in as sensitive a way as possible', and realise that this seemed rather enigmatic to some. I (as the geneticist) was not proposing a solution to the dilemma, but outlining what I would do in practice, faced with the prospect of Jane undergoing prophylactic surgery. I still think in such a situation, Phyllis's confidentiality ought to be breached, but that if Jane guessed the provenance of the information, I should not confirm this. I liked Hurwitz's approach to this: 'If forced mediation fails, the issue should be fudged and Jane offered the genetic test but without divulging the source of the genetic information. This subterfuge would avoid a formal and transparent breach of Phyllis's confidentiality, and would allow surgery to be avoided if Jane proves BRCA-gene negative'. GMC and BMA guidelines suggest that if a breach is to be made it should be made explicit to Phyllis, but I would argue that to not do so (in this case) causes the least harm to both parties. I accept that Jane is likely to infer that the information comes from Phyllis but I would state that I am not at liberty to confirm and imply, if questioned directly, that it could have come from a variety of sources (e.g. contact with Great Uncle Stan in Australia). The dilemma thus remains unresolved but it would be my preferred practical solution in an acute situation. I accept of course Hurwitz's point that 'the narrator may exercise determinative influences on how we respond to the dilemma described'.

Although I would agree with Savulescu in favour of disclosure, I would not argue this on the basis of benefit to Jane's daughters and future daughters. Her existing daughters are still young and at least one or two decades away from being at risk of either breast or ovarian cancer. Much can happen in the way of preventative options, diagnosis or treatment in this time. To argue that a child should not be born because they might develop breast or ovarian cancer as an adult, seems to me a step too far. Very few people harbouring a BRCA1 mutation have opted for prenatal diagnosis in a pregnancy, although the techniques would now be standard and accurate. Furthermore, it may yet be proven that BRCA1 mutation carriers are at a huge advantage for some other aspect of life – maybe they are less susceptible to, say, flu or heart disease.

Concluding comments

There is no consensus among the chapters in this book on a resolution to this case (we are not helped by Jane Austen: 'Where an opinion is general, it is usually correct.'). Or, as Withers writes, 'the "end" will point me in more than one direction'. The dilemma remains, even if we chose one particular outcome. The author of the scenario may decide to breach confidentiality in *this* case but it does not mean she has sided with Jane or has no sympathy with Phyllis, or that she would do the same if the case was subtly different.

Many professionals in clinical genetics have little training or knowledge in ethics. In cases such as the one described in this book, they may search in vain for clarifying guidelines or clear legal statements to help them. The chapters in this book offer perceptive and intelligent insights to the case. By examining the case from many different angles and perspectives, they help to dispel the confusion and bewilderment that professionals dealing with such a dilemma may experience.

REFERENCES

Brose, M. S., Rebbeck, T. R., Calzone, K. A. *et al.* (2002). Cancer risk estimates for BRCA1 mutation carriers identified in a risk evaluation program. *J Natl Cancer Inst*, **94**, 1365–72.

Clarke, A. (1991). Is non-directive genetic counselling possible? *Lancet*, **338**(8773), 998–1001.

Frost, M. H., Schaid, D. J., Sellers, T. A. *et al.* (2000). Long-term satisfaction and psychological and social function following bilateral prophylactic mastectomy. *JAMA*, **284**(3), 319–24.

Haber, D. (2002). Prophylactic oophorectomy to reduce the risk of ovarian and breast cancer in carriers of BRCA mutations. *N Engl J Med*, **346**(21), 1660–2.

Hartmann, L. C., Schaid, D. J., Woods, J. E. *et al.* (1999). Efficacy of bilateral prophylactic mastectomy in women with a family history of breast cancer. *N Engl J Med*, **340**(2), 77–84.

Human Genetics Commission. (2002). *Inside Information Balancing Interests in the Use of Personal Genetic Data.* (May). London.

Julian-Reynier, C., Eisinger, F., Chabal, F. *et al.* (2000). Disclosure to the family of breast/ovarian cancer genetic test results: patient's willingness and associated factors. *Am J Med Gen*, **94**(1), 13–18.

Kauff, N. D., Satagopan, J. M., Robson, M. E. *et al.* (2002). Risk-reducing salpingo-oophorectomy in women with BRCA1 or BRCA2 mutation. *N Engl J Med*, **346**(21), 1609–15.

Lucassen, A. M. and Parker, M. (2001). Talking about paternity in the genetic clinic: some ethical considerations. *Lancet*, **357**, 1033–5.

Lucassen, A. M., Watson, E. W. and Eccles, D. (2001). Management of a young woman with a family history of breast cancer. *BMJ*, **322**, 1040–2.

Meijers-Heijboer, H., van Geel, B., van Putten, W. L. *et al.* (2001). Breast cancer after prophylactic bilateral mastectomy in women with a BRCA1 or BRCA2 mutation. *N Engl J Med*, **345**(3), 159–64.

Meijers-Heijboer, E. J., Brohet, R. M., Asperen, C. J. *et al.* (2004). Risks of cancer at sites other than breast and ovary among BRCA1 mutation carriers. *Familial Cancer*, abstr.

Morrow, M. and Gradishar, W. (2002). Breast cancer. *BMJ*, **324**(7334), 410–14.

Rebbeck, T. R., Lynch, H. T., Neuhausen, S. L. *et al.* (2002). Prophylactic oophorectomy in carriers of BRCA1 or BRCA2 mutations. *N Engl J Med*, **346**(21), 1616–22.

Thompson, D. and Easton, D. F. (2002). Breast cancer linkage consortium: cancer incidence in BRCA1 mutation carriers. *J Natl Cancer Inst*, **94**(18), 1358–65.

15

Philosophical reflections

Michael Parker, Richard Ashcroft, Marian Verkerk,
Guy Widdershoven

In the centre of Fedora, that grey stone metropolis, stands a metal building with a
crystal globe in every room. Looking into each globe, you see a blue city, a model of
a different Fedora. These are the forms the city could have taken if, for one reason
or another, it had not become what we see today. In every age someone, looking at
Fedora as it was, imagined a way of making it the ideal city, but while he
constructed his miniature model, Fedora was already no longer the same as before,
and what had until yesterday a possible future became only a toy in a glass globe.

(Calvino 1972).

Much writing and thinking in bioethics takes the form of a kind of
Calvinesque speculative architecture. Our aim in this book and in the particular way in which it has been created has been to do something different. We
wanted, in particular, to encourage the contributors to engage with one
another and with the case to a degree unusual in bioethics practice. Behind
this intention is something like a commitment to the idea that moral
development, the growth of moral understanding and the emergence of
moral practice in medicine (and in bioethics) can be facilitated by
encouraging moral philosophers and health professionals to engage with
one another in a focused and reasonably structured setting. More broadly it
is to argue that conversation is a developmental fundamental of human
experience (Parker 1995). This is not to suggest that under certain formal
conversational conditions 'consensus' or some kind of 'moral truth' will
naturally or inevitably emerge.

First, the approach adopted here, in the creation of this text, was
informal. The deliberations we engaged in were not structured according
to explicit deliberative rules: we just talked to each other. Of course, there
are implicit cultural and other rules permeating the way we related to one
another but essentially the authors simply got together, presented their
ideas, gathered up comments from the other authors and the editorial
team and then, in the peace of their own offices (or on the bus), pursued

Case Analysis in Clinical Ethics, ed. Richard Ashcroft, Anneke Lucassen, Michael Parker,
Marian Verkerk, Guy Widdershoven. Published by Cambridge University Press.

the ideas that occurred to them in these conversations as best they could and as far as they would take them.

Second, just as the idea that intersubjective deliberation (or conversation) is central to the growth of understanding need not imply that such conversation must conform to explicit rules, neither does it imply any claim about the objective truth of the resulting understandings, nor still that the authors or readers of this text will come to understand things in the same way. Of course, there is implicit in all of this an assumption that those engaged in the conversation are either able to bring to the table a shared language sufficient for conversation to begin, or able once there to find ways to develop such a language or languages. But this is not to claim very much: human beings do this all the time. On reflection, perhaps this is to claim a very great deal. Even so, it does happen. Having written that deliberation need not require rules, it is, of course, immediately obvious that this is not the case at all. The effectiveness and indeed the enjoyment of these workshops was made possible by warmth, mutual respect, openness, a willingness to listen to and to offer critical comments, a commitment to the giving of and listening to reasons, combined with a shared interest in the broad intention to create a bioethics book in a new way. And all of this took place against a background of shared cultural, academic and other assumptions about the way in which life is to be lived and conversations to be had. There is not much that can be done about this. In any case, it worked for us.

As always, aims and objectives emerge after the event to some extent. Our initial aims were (fairly) modest. They were to write a book in bioethics exemplifying in a single volume the different and contrasting ways in which bioethicists from different perspectives and countries respond when invited to engage with a single case. One of our aims was to show the reader the way the mind of a bioethicist works, at its best. In a way it is quite surprising that no one has done this before. Most books on bioethics (before this one) seem to have taken one of the following three forms. One type of approach introduces the subject by presenting the reader with a series of chapters on 'key themes' in bioethics such as 'end of life', 'confidentiality', 'medical research' and so on. Another sets before the consumer a smorgasbord of contrasting methodological approaches to bioethics, exhibiting such delicacies as 'utilitarian ethics', the 'four principles' and 'narrative ethics'. Sometimes single-author texts on bioethics do address a single theme, such as, for example, medical research, and set out to explain what different perspectives in bioethics might have to say about the theme. But our aim in this volume was to encourage bioethicists from different perspectives to engage with one another and with a health professional in the exploration of the ethical dimensions of a realistic and intricate case and to contrast their approaches by showing them at work, on the same case, in a single volume.

The case

Although it is realistic and based in clinical reality, the case used in this book is, of course, a construct created for a particular purpose or range of purposes (Chambers 1999). The constructedness of the case is not concealed, however. It is in this respect a case *after* Richard Rogers (to pursue the architectural metaphor) – with all the workings on the outside. (Richard Rogers is the British architect who designed the Pompidou Centre in Paris, among other well-known buildings, famous for designs revealing the internal 'machinery' of the buildings he creates.) Notwithstanding its constructedness, the case is rich and recognisable both to clinicians and family members and, for the reader, we hope it offers in its combination with the other chapters the possibility of a kind of bioethical flight-simulator.

Most 'case-based' works in bioethics are not in fact case-based at all in any sense that clinicians or patients would recognise. Whether in the form of books or academic papers, bioethics writing tends to use very short, (usually less than half a page), abstract(ed) 'case studies' (whether real or hypothetical) chosen, or created, for a particular purpose. That is, as seed crystals around which a bioethics publication can be grown. In this respect Todd Chambers' critique of case-based bioethics is pertinent. These cases tend to be hyperconstructed or perhaps overreduced. The case in this book is not short but it is constructed. We hope however that our construction is sensitive to the environment and ecofriendly.

What is different about our case? First, the case we use is chapter length. This is unusual, if not unique. Second, it is written by a clinician working every day with these kinds of cases. So, whilst the case is hypothetical it is based on and is an elaboration of the real and complicated world of clinical practice. There are conflicts, confusions and voids. This is as it should be as a case like this would be experienced in practice. The case has, we think, the feel of the real about it (whatever that means).

Anyway, as the chapters show, it certainly pushed the bioethicists into real, hard thought – the kind of thought that is only possible with messy and complicated cases. Cases, that is, that refuse to lie down and take their bioethical medicine. In addition to its initial creation by Anneke Lucassen, a further dimension to the case's constructedness lies in the fact that the initial version was circulated to the bioethicist editors, early on in the process, in order to make sure that it was suited to its literary and philosophical purpose. For this, the case had to have sufficient detail and nuance to be able to give something for the bioethicists and the readers to get their teeth into. In response to Anneke's first version of the case the other editors made comments like 'there isn't enough of a story for the narrative ethicist to be able to say anything useful' or 'could you give us a bit more about the problematic relationship between Jane and Phyllis?'

or 'we don't understand why you couldn't just test her directly'. In the light of comments such as these, and some further questions about aspects of the genetics and clinical practice, Anneke rewrote (reconstructed) the case.

But this was not the end of the reconstruction. The process of writing the book subsequently involved sending the case to each of the invited authors and asking them to write draft versions of their chapters. These draft versions were then presented at four workshops where they were discussed with Anneke, the other editors and two or three other authors. This led to some further modifications of the case. A final version was produced by Anneke after her final reading of the final versions of the chapters. So, the case has a life of its own and has in many ways outgrown the chapters it spawned. The case has been growing in relation to its bioethical environment, so too the chapters and the thoughts of the bioethicists in their relation to the case and to a clinician.

Method

The original idea of inviting the authors to present their chapters at workshops, rather than simply requiring them to be submitted for a deadline in the usual way, was to provide them and the editors with an opportunity to comment on how the draft versions might be developed into final chapters and to provide the authors with an opportunity to clarify their understanding of the case and the clinical details with Anneke. In the end, however, the workshops became much more than this and the writing of the book ended up taking an organic form of its own. Perhaps surprisingly, this has not led to greater homogeneity between the forms of the chapters. In fact, if anything, the chapters have become more distinct. The fact that each of the chapters has been subject to a kind of informal deliberation has, we think, enriched them in their diversity, and certainly enriched for all of us the process of contributing to the book. In the end, the different methods adopted by each of the authors became more rather than less important, despite the fact that the book did evolve into a form of multidisciplinary writing enterprise. Nevertheless, whilst consensus was not reached on what to do in the case, something like agreement was reached on the idea that conversation between the various perspectives added something to each of them. What seemed to emerge in the end was not a resolution of the case, or of questions such as, for example, those about moral realism versus relativism, but a keen awareness that at the heart of moral action is something like good judgement, in the light of engaged deliberation.

The starting point for writing this book, and in the end one of its conclusions too, was a belief in the importance of method, of the distinct but interrelated ways in which we (as bioethicists, patients and clinicians) make sense of the moral world in which we live and practice and the philosophical, intellectual and emotional tools we use to do so. Even if in the end we come to similar decisions about what to do in a particular situation, we each see the moral landscape surrounding the situation or decision differently. It makes sense to us in ways that differ. We would give different justifications and reasons in different ways. This is as important as the decision we make, or would make. And, of course, those who chose similarly in this case, would diverge in their views in other cases. Each of the methodologies on display here would be required to choose differently from one another under certain conditions. The aim of the book, therefore, is broader than the resolution of a particular case. Indeed, this book is not in the end about a single case nor still about genetics. This is the story of one family, one limited technology and of a particular time. Other families will be different. Technology around genetic testing will develop and it will soon be possible to test without requiring the mutational analysis from another family member. But this is not the point. The aim of the book is not to provide a multiperspectival consideration of a particular problem, although it does that, but to show how bioethicists work the *chiaroscuro* of bioethics in relation to healthcare practice.

Values

Each of the writers is committed to her or his method (or committed enough to write a chapter on it at least). Why is this? Why do people choose one method rather than another? Why do some people adopt a more consequent-ialist approach? Why are some people attracted to principles, some to narratives? These are not questions that can be answered here but they are important questions for anyone reading a book such as this to consider. The perspectives chosen must in some ways relate to the authors' values and beliefs and there must of course also be influences related to gender, culture and so on at work. In addition to an awareness of the values and beliefs leading bioethicists to adopt one perspective rather than another, a reader of this volume (and any other like it) needs also to be aware that the range of perspectives chosen by the editors itself constitutes a selection from a very wide range of possible perspectives. What would a Buddhist bioethicist, or a bioethicist from a developing country make of all of this? Why did we choose the authors and the perspective we did rather than others? This is a good question. Certainly our intention with this book was not to provide a comprehensive survey of bioethics, nor was it intended to be a selection of the best perspectives, suggesting that perspectives not included are of lesser value. We had to stop somewhere and we stopped where we did.

To what extent does diversity matter? One approach to thinking about bioethics would be to say that what is important in bioethics are the arguments used, the analysis of the validity of those arguments and the truth of their constituent empirical premises. On this account, it does not matter *why* someone makes a particular argument. What is of central importance, from this perspective, is the question of whether the argument, say, for example, in favour of respecting Phyllis's confidentiality, stands up to scrutiny. This is one way of thinking about bioethics but it would be a strange position to take, if one meant it literally, for none of the arguments and reasons elaborated in these chapters or any other arguments anywhere would make any sense at all except in the context of linguistic, social and cultural forms of life. While reasons and arguments are indeed extremely powerful and important linguistic, emotional and intellectual forms of language and features of the way in which we live and speak to each other, this is precisely because of their embeddedness in human forms of life, not because of their independence from them. While a certain degree of 'independence' is necessary to the ability to be able to reason and argue, this does not require and could not require one to cease to be human. Moral reasons, problems and arguments have the force for us that they do only by virtue of the fact that we live in a world with others. This, indeed, is why it is so important for us to get clear about the reasons we have for doing one thing rather than another when confronted by a case such as the one involving Phyllis and Jane.

Real people, real lives

In the end, the arguments in this book concern real people's lives, even if indirectly. Even though the case itself is a hypothetical and constructed fiction, the fact is that there are people walking in to genetics clinics around the world, on a daily basis, who are having to face the question of whether and how information about their genetic make-up should be shared with their relatives. The things that bioethicists say about bioethics and healthcare practice are ultimately comments about the moral dimensions of the lives of real people at difficult times in their lives. Health professionals such as Anneke have the privilege to encounter people at these key moments in the human condition: pregnancy, birth, death, loss and so on. Bioethics too is concerned, at its best, with how to live, how to decide and how to relate to people at these key moments. This requires us to take our job seriously. It also requires us to try our best (at least sometimes) to be more engaged with the ethical issues arising in the lives of real people (whether health professionals or patients) than the *Fedorese* are in their approach to architecture.

REFERENCES

Calvino, I. (1972). *Invisible Cities*. London: Picador.
Chambers, T. (1999). *The Fiction of Bioethics: Cases as Literary Texts*. New York: Routledge.
Parker, M. (1995). *The Growth of Understanding*. Aldershot: Avebury.

Index